The Glass Between Us

Eileen Rudnick

The Glass Between Us

Eileen Rudnick

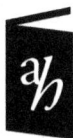

Apprentice House
Baltimore, Maryland

Printed in the United States of America

First Edition

Cover Photo by Julie Sayo
Back Cover Photo by Michael Paul Rudnick

Published by Apprentice House
The Future of Publishing...Today!

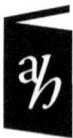

Apprentice House
Communication Department
Loyola University Maryland
4501 N. Charles Street
Baltimore, MD 21210

410.617.5265
410.617.2198 fax
www.ApprenticeHouse.com
info@ApprenticeHouse.com

To Mike, the foundation of my recovery, with love.

Table of Contents

Prologue

Before you turn to page one and begin reading, I want you to consider the possibility of becoming disabled today. I know that it is more common to imagine the consequences of unexpected death. Questions like, "Is there life after death?" and "What will happen to my family?" may come to mind. But suppose you don't quite die? You may survive a near-death experience and emerge irrevocably changed, having lost a part of you but not all of you. What then?

I began writing this book when I was less than five years out of coma, starting with Chapter 1. I am now almost ten years beyond the motor vehicle collision that was my rebirth. And even though my writing skills have improved, I have not rewritten any of the early chapters. Each one stands as testimony to my growth and recovery.

The odyssey begins with my extraordinary near-death vision, continues with emergence from coma, through the years of rehabilitation and growth, and ends in my current new life. All the while, the Kubler-Ross five stages of grief (denial, anger, bargaining, depression, and acceptance) will be apparent.

Don't assume that this is a two-hankie book. It is not. You will cry, but you will also laugh. You will experience not only anger, but also gratification. And in the end, you will be uplifted.

Eileen Rudnick
June 2010

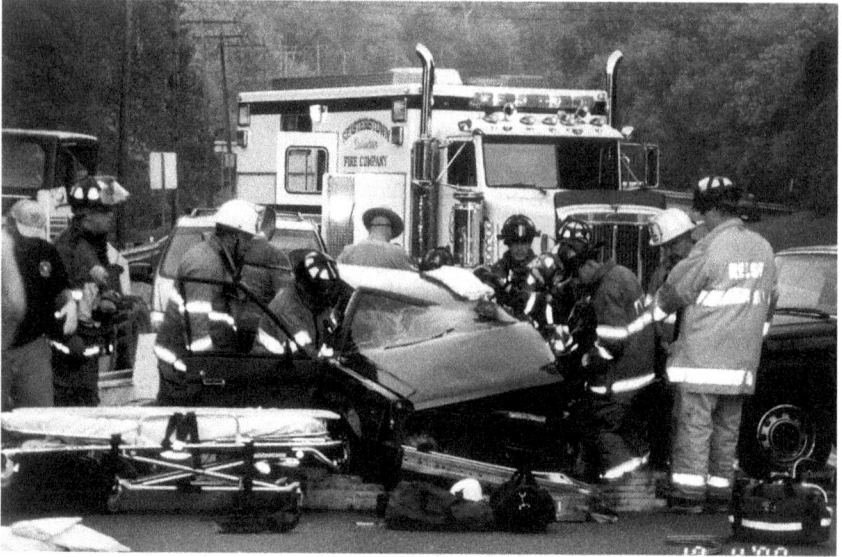

My car was reduced in size by about one third, and paramedics worked to extricate me.

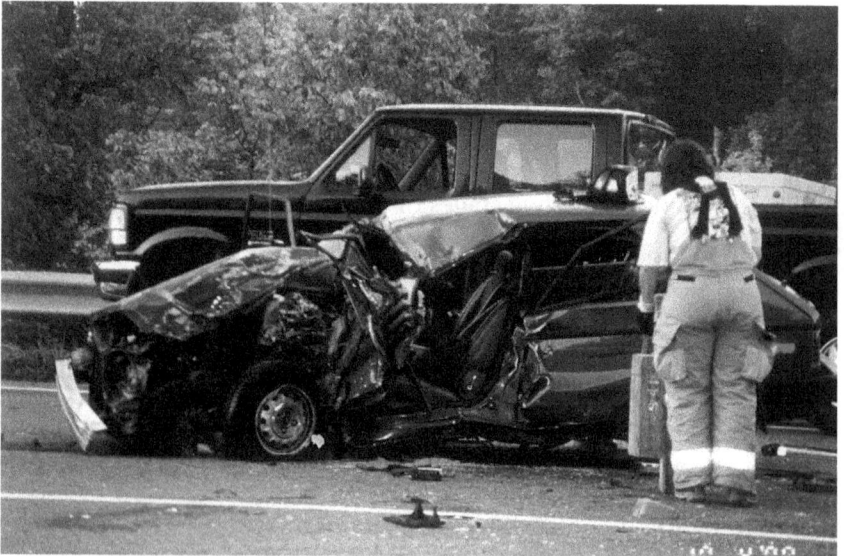

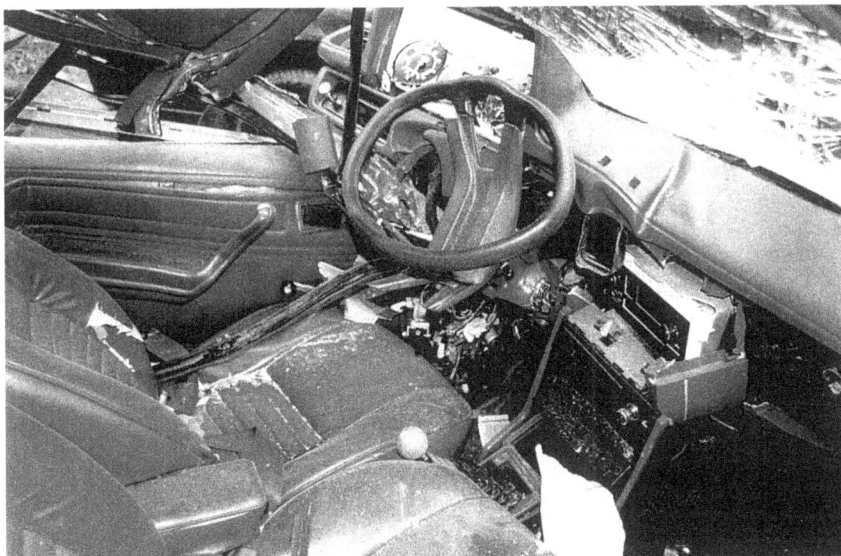

I was taken for a short ride to the medivac helicopter that had landed in a field about two miles away.

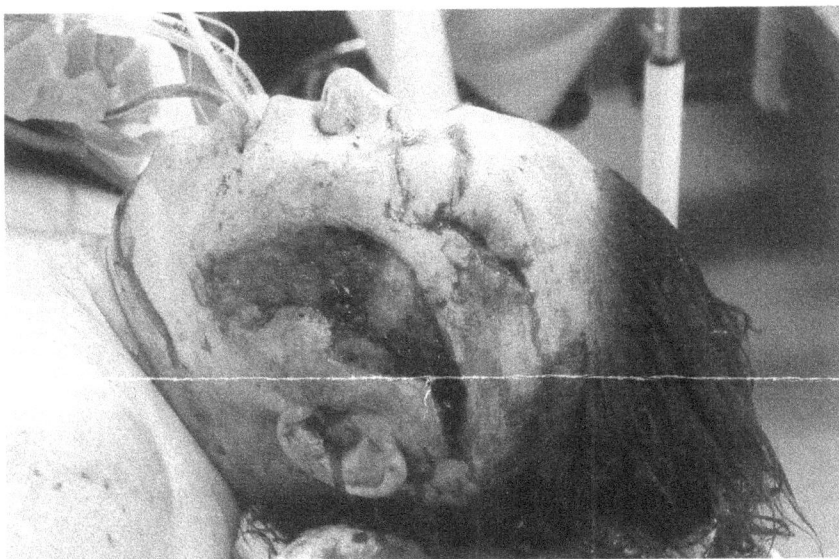

I was swollen and lacerated beyond recognition. My left eye socket was shattered, and my ear was displaced toward the back of my head.

I Am Not Alone...

❑ Do you have sudden, overwhelming fatigue even on an average day?

❑ Do you have trouble starting or completing projects?

❑ Do you have trouble understanding conversations, whether or not you are included?

❑ Do you constantly re-read instructions or have them repeated?

❑ Does it seem like your body sensations don't make sense according to your environment? Maybe your left and right sides' sensations don't match.

❑ Do you struggle to remember what you were doing? Where you were going? Whether or not you've eaten? The telephone call you've just finished?

❑ Do you tend to be too emotional? Too angry? Hypersensitive? Cry easily?

❑ Is your speech slower than average and less fluent because words are not easy to find?

❑ Is solving problems a challenge for you?

❑ Is your behavior not socially acceptable? Do you stand too close? Are you sometimes out of control?

❑ Are you subject to seizures?

❑ Do you have unexplained clumsiness?

- ❑ Do you avoid responsibility?

- ❑ Do you get stuck on one subject, like a broken record?

- ❑ Are you too impulsive?

- ❑ Do you have much more or much less interest in sex?

- ❑ Is reading comprehension difficult?

- ❑ Are your senses giving you more vivid or less vivid messages?

- ❑ Do you have a sleep disorder?

- ❑ Does your self-esteem depend upon the opinions of others?

- ❑ Do you have marked sensitivity to medication? Alcohol?

- ❑ Do you feel apart from everyone? Different?

- ❑ Do friends and relatives tell you that you are not yourself?

- ❑ Can stress make it very hard to think?

- ❑ Do you have holes in your memory?

- ❑ Do you have double or obstructed vision? Always? Sometimes?

- ❑ Is your hearing not clear? Does your name have to be called more than once?

- ❑ Do you have restless limbs? Do they tingle and jump?

- ❑ Do you feel like you are not completely toilet trained?

- ❑ Do you have poor judgment?

- ❑ Is your gait changed? Unreliable? Need a wheelchair? A cane?

❑ Do you have chronic pain? Severe headaches?

❑ Are you jumpy, nervous, and easily startled?

❑ Are your dark moods more intense? Are you plagued by depression?

❑ Is your spiritual life more meaningful?

❑ Do you feel like you've had another life?

❑ Do you feel like stranger lives in your body?

If you can answer "yes" to some or to many of these questions, and you couldn't before, you may have acquired a brain injury. It is not a terminal illness, but it is a chronic condition.

Lost...

"Is all that we see or seem but a dream within a dream?"
-Edgar Allan Poe

Coma

I watched from a distance as she walked toward me. Her progress was unhurried. I seemed to be standing still but I was not sure because I did not feel anything under my feet. The surrounding soft, green light captured my attention. We were in a garden, the likes of which is not seen, except in dreams. Exceedingly tall plants grew up around us, some topped with vivid blossoms, far out of reach. The woman and I existed at root level, like ants. There was only peace and beauty in this quiet place and I could feel a smile of pleasure well up inside me. The verdant scent reminded me of pleasurable moments in my grandfather's garden, lying on my back between the rows. I felt warm, safe, and secure - one with the plants. Within the garden was sanctuary from a troubled childhood. Precisely spaced stalks of corn touched the sky; there was a hedgerow of lacy carrot tops, and determined green peas drooped with the weight of heavy pods. A clean, wet baby carrot was a childhood favorite, in addition to a pocketful of pea pods, still warm from the sun. Gentle chiding from Grandpa was not scary like the more harsh punishment I would have received from my father. Yearly, my sisters and I reveled in a blissful two-week holiday with our loving Granny and Grandpa in their peaceful and simple home. I loved the statuesque hollyhocks that stood together in the corner, like grand dames in colorful gowns.

However, I felt pain that seemed to be everywhere -- as if I had been beaten. Then I was viewing a scene from years ago at that scary row house in the city of Montreal. I was a child and in the back room off the kitchen. I was scared because Mummy and Daddy were mad. They were yelling at each other. He hit her hard on the face to shut her up but she just screamed louder. I put my hands over my ears because I wanted her to be quiet, too. Maybe then, he would just go back out to the bar, and we would not have to see him again until tomorrow. My two sisters, one younger, one older, sneaked in from the back yard and we huddled together, silently, in the back room, hoping that Mummy and Daddy would not notice us. No Luck! Before long, my fear turned to near panic because Daddy was staggering from the front room through the kitchen calling the names of my older sister and me. We were in trouble because he found out about the papers we had touched when he told us not to. He grabbed my sister first and demanded to know why we did it. Her terrified screams echoed my mother's screams. Mummy tried to get her away from Daddy but he pushed her away, while clutching a fistful of my sister's hair. Mummy fell on her backside while Daddy hit my sister as hard as he could across the face more than once. They were both hysterical and I hated the sound of the punches. I gazed with pity at the five year old hugging herself and staring at the wall. She knew that she was next but the wait was torturous. I knew her thoughts; she was determined not to cry because it just made Daddy worse. When his hard hand closed around her boney arm, jerking her to her feet, she wet her pants. The blows to her face and body took her breath away but she endured it in silence. In the end, she was proud because she did not cry. She was ashamed of her wet clothes, though, and hoped that she would not wet the bed again that night.

As I watched the naked five year old clean up her own pee, while enduring her mother's ridicule, the scene changed and I turned my attention back to the woman in the garden. The light, chestnut-brown hair, greenish eyes, and freckled skin were very familiar. She was small, but womanly. When her sunny regard washed over me I was excited to acknowledge the presence of my restored mother. This youthful, vibrant woman is proof of what will happen to me upon my death, I thought. My mind, body, and soul will be reunited when I die. Moreover, even if some of the parts are broken, damaged, or diseased, the sum of my whole person will be fresh and new. I know this to be true because my mother had died three years previously, withered, with a few tufts of white hair and delirious from morphine for the pain of cancer. This must be how she looked in her youth, which I don't remember.

Reality

On another level, the trauma team moved quickly and expertly over the mangled mess of a woman lying helplessly unconscious before them. The torn and bloodied mess of my favorite green dress was lying on the floor by the gurney with the rest of my clothing that had been cut from my body. I had arrived by helicopter moments before, after being extracted from a twisted wreck. Just one hour ago I had been driving home from work. Now my life was on hold and my survival in question. The excitement of my new job with a significant raise in salary was already over and I would never return.

I have searched my injured brain very hard to locate my absolute last memory before the trauma. I think it is as follows: It was approximately twelve hours before the collision (6am) and I was viewing my reflection in the mirror over my dresser. My favorite emerald green earrings sparkled nicely in my ears and I was attempting to pin up some of my medium length, thick, reddish brown hair. I remember cursing it, wishing that I had gotten it cut, because it was taking too much time to deal with. My dress was hunter green and I loved wearing it. I thought that I had all my best days when I wore that dress because I felt utterly confident. Once again, I noted that it would be good to lose thirty pounds. As I tied my brand new tennis shoes, which I used for driving, I thought with unknown irony that if I was in an accident that day at least all my undergarments were new. I lost the earrings, the dress, the new shoes, the new undergarments, my hair, and thirty pounds. I gained a brain injury, scars, and deformities. I have concluded that it would have been an unforgettable day, if not for the amnesia.

Suicide Hill

The Emergency Medical Services (EMS) team from Reese Volunteer Fire Company in Carroll County, Maryland arrived at the scene (Route 140 and Old Gamber Road) of a reported three-car collision at about 6:20pm on a mild Tuesday evening in early October. What they found was a black SUV impacted with a small, older, red car, which had been completely demolished. The SUV was not badly damaged, so there must be another vehicle involved.

Witnesses at the scene pointed to a white pickup truck stopped against the guardrail about 500 feet away and facing in the wrong direction.

The desolate, but uninjured young driver sat on the guard rail, having been shooed away by arriving police from trying desperately to help the dying woman in the car. Meanwhile, the also uninjured SUV driver, who was more concerned about finding a way out of possible litigation, was rehearsing the story he was going to tell.

The EMS team captain, Sam Mann, assessed my condition at the scene. He reported an unconscious female with a compound fracture of the left arm, facial lacerations, compressed chest, Glasgow Coma Scale (GCS) 5, shallow respirations of 6 to 8, and tachycardia. A helicopter was summoned and arrived before the extraction was complete. The rescue team had me out of the wreck in about 20 minutes, though. The trickiest part, it turned out, was freeing my left foot, which was wedged under the driver's side door. The entire car had been compressed by about one third on the driver's side and on top. The roof had been crushed downward. My small size was a factor in my survival. I later thanked them for not giving up, which would have been easier. The last assessment of my condition by Sam Mann indicated that I was combative, made unintelligible sounds, and had developed bluish skin and raccoon eyes. Later, when I was at Reese Fire Station to thank them, I asked about the meaning of raccoon eyes. They told me that when a patient is near death, a sunken, dark-ringed look appears around the eyes. The helicopter ride to R Adams Cowley Shock Trauma (Shock Trauma) at University of Maryland Medical Center (UMMC) took eight minutes; the one-hour ambulance ride would have gotten me there "too late", according to Dr. Carnell Cooper, trauma specialist.

My worried husband, awaiting my arrival at home, was making desperate phone calls. In one heartbreaking moment, Mike learned from the state police in Westminster that his wife had been transported to Shock Trauma, priority one, but not expected to live. My terrified family rushed to UMMC with the worst expectation. My Mike had to endure the horror of identifying the still alive Jane Doe on the trauma unit. He was shown a mangled, swollen mass, bandaged and bundled. Mike has told me that all he could see was some of my reddish-brown hair sticking straight up at the top of my head through the bandages. When he was handed my wedding ring and a nurse kindly lifted the lid of my one good eye, he knew it was I.

This is from my husband, Mike, in answer to my question about his memory of the day of the accident. My interview with him was highly emotional for both of us. Mike's account reveals that his trauma is still fresh. His recall has holes in it (on purpose), and he has difficulty with sequencing.

> We had only one car, and you drove to work
> after dropping me off. I worked during the day at
> Springfield Hospital Center and got a ride home. I
> had a scratchy throat, so I did not work at Wal-Mart.
> I was home a little while, and then you called and
> said that you were going to be late and what time you
> were leaving work. I knew the route, having shown
> it to you, and I knew how long it took to get home.

*About the time you were due home, I began to worry.
Then I continued to worry more and more because it
was starting to get dark. About 25 minutes after you
were due home, I called your office, and there was no
answer. So I waited some more, watched the news,
and did not see anything, and still no word. My two
basic fears were A) You had an accident and B) You
were abducted somehow. So then, I looked in the
phone book, and called the Baltimore County police
that covered the Hunt Valley area. I asked if there
had been an accident and they said no. Then I called
the State Police in Westminster. They asked my name
and told me to hold on a minute. When they came
back, they told me to sit down. They said that you
were in a bad accident, that it did not look good, and
that you were being flown to Shock Trauma. I called
Beth (our daughter.) She was already on her way,
because I called earlier to borrow her car to go look
for you. When she arrived, I called Mike (our son)
and told him that you had an accident and were on
your way to Shock Trauma. I could go into details
about pacing, worrying, watching TV and praying,
but that is what happened.*

The following is Mike's response to my question about his
thoughts and feelings at that crucial time.

About an hour went by after you were due home.
The feeling was similar to the one when you are
waiting for your kid to get home. With you, it was

different, though, because you were always on time. If there were a reason to be late, you would have called me. I did not think that you were going to die. I do not know why. Maybe it is a faith issue or my nursing background. The drive to Shock Trauma felt different from the drive to Baltimore County Hospital when my Dad died. I knew he was dead before I got there. I knew the situation was serious and the State Police said that you probably were not going to make it but I did!

This is Mike's answer to, "What happened when you got to Shock Trauma?" Please note that he mentions a sign of severe brain injury - thrashing.

Mike was already there (he lived in Baltimore.) Beth and I had time to comfort each other on the drive to the hospital but Mike was frantically trying to get in to see you. I gave them my name and in a few moments, they took me to see you. You were wrapped in a sheet like a mummy and your head was wrapped. It was very hard to recognize you. You kept trying to move your left leg. I still think that it was because the car had a clutch and maybe you were still trying to press it. I could only recognize you because of your eyes. I asked about your wedding ring. They had removed it but they gave it to me. Dr. Cooper said that there was internal bleeding and that they had to do surgery right away. You had other injuries but that was the most life threatening. I went back downstairs and let the kids know. I stayed with them and tried to be strong for them. My sister and her husband were there but they left soon. I did not think that you were going to die. I do not know why. Your one eye was open. I just had a feeling. You were young and in good health.

Then I asked, (Was I looking at you, was I making any noise, and was I moving anything besides my left leg?)

Not that I remember. It has been over 5 years. I sound calm now but I was not then. I was scared and I have tried to forget. I would like to talk about your eyes being open.

They were actually pulled open. Your green eyes told me it was you. Your general appearance was swollen. You looked heavier and I am sure that was because of the internal bleeding. Even though you were wrapped in a sheet or blanket, your torso seemed heavier. You might have moved your head a little bit but they were trying to keep your head still. There were no restraints and you were not on life-support yet. I could not tell if you were looking at anything. I recognized you because of your green eyes but one was swelling shut. You did not make any noise. I could tell that you were in discomfort and I tried to reassure you. The staff around you was also trying to reassure you. You were listed as a Jane Doe so I had to positively identify you. Dr. Cooper listed your injuries but the staff at Shock Trauma was very calm and professional. They were objective and did not comment about your condition.

Dr. Carnell Cooper made a careful examination of my unconscious form noting my numerous injuries. They were as follows: pelvic fracture, internal hemorrhage, collapsed lung (which showed signs of pneumonia, later), compound fracture of the left arm, torn and blocked blood vessels of the left arm, dislocated left shoulder, left scapula fracture, serious soft tissue damage to my left face, assorted skull and facial fractures, and brain injury. He gave me a GCS score of 8 or 9, which indicated a moderate to severe injury. Dr. Cooper was very concerned about the evident internal hemorrhage, especially when my blood pressure became unstable; therefore, he had me in emergency surgery within an hour of my arrival. He successfully found and repaired liver lacerations, thanks to the argon laser. The lacerations were more like deep punctures in a cushion, and situated very awkwardly on the back of the liver. I survived in spite of the significant loss of blood. I did not awaken after surgery, however, because I remained in a coma for about five days and I would never be the same. Dr. Cooper will always be Superman to me and to my family.

More from my interview with Mike (Tell me about your time at Shock Trauma until you were finally able to go home.)

It was a few hours before your first surgery was over and then I got another call from Dr. Cooper. You had a very bad liver laceration, but they used an argon laser to repair it. He said that without it you would have bled to death. He said that what they actually did was open your abdomen and quarter you with packing to find out where the bleeding was. He assured me that no other organs were damaged and that they had stopped the bleeding. He said that he called in Dr. Andy Eglseder to look at your left arm and that you had extensive damage to your face and skull. There was no mention of brain injury at that time but Dr. Cooper said that there was no cerebral bleeding.

While my scared and desperate family watched and waited, I continued to spend time in an enchanted garden with my late mother. As she came close to me, I marveled at the strong resemblance between us. We did not touch. Instead, my mother extended her slim hand toward me in a gesture not to come any closer. She said with strength and conviction, "You can't stay. You have to go back. You still have too much work to do."

I do not know if I answered but that was the end of our time together. My husband has reported to me that one of my earliest queries when I became conscious was, which hospital room did my mother have. I still wonder if I am accomplishing the work that she mentioned.

I have no memory of the time I spent at Shock Trauma, and I carry a lot of guilt with me because of what my family endured on my account. They watched a bruised, deformed, and unfamiliar version of me struggle for survival on life support. Then they watched as I endured four surgeries in five days, while still in a coma. My family has told me that the brief visit they were given with me was suddenly ended because Dr. Cooper did not like the look of my arm and was afraid that I would lose it without immediate surgery. Dr. Andy Eglseder, Orthopaedic Specialist, to repair my left arm, performed the second surgery. Both bones in my forearm were fractured. The compound fracture was fixed with a titanium rod screwed onto each bone. As I write this, I am stroking my left arm, feeling the titanium through the skin. As long as I do not put excessive pressure on the sight, carry extra heavy loads, or twist my arm repeatedly, there is no discomfort. Dr. Eglseder also had to restore normal blood flow; I had been without a pulse in my left arm since the collision. He located the torn and blocked blood vessels, made careful repairs, tested the restored blood flow, and saved my arm, which now works beautifully. It is straight and, except for the scars, does not have the appearance of having been nearly lost. My remembered meetings with Dr. Eglseder were like being with a cheerful neighbor and friend. I have wondered how he stays so positive in the midst of all the human body destruction he sees.

> (Mike) Dr. Cooper told me that there was no pulse in your left arm. There were fractures, and there was vascular damage. I talked to Dr. Eglseder and gave him permission to do surgery. Therefore, I went downstairs and told the kids to go and get some rest. About one or two in the morning I saw Dr. Eglseder, who described how they repaired your arm. He said that the blood vessels had been repaired and that you

now had good blood flow to your hand.

I had seen you in the madhouse of the TRU (Trauma Resuscitation Unit) a few times but they were going to move you to a room. I asked if I could get the kids in to see you. I am 90% sure of this but it has been over 5 years and I have really tried to forget, so my facts may not be as good as perhaps I would like them to be. I had sent the kids to Mike's to get some rest earlier but they were back by then. It was about 2 am and you were in your first living quarters. Everyone was talking aloud but you were not very responsive. You might have squeezed a hand, but that was all. You had one big accident and two surgeries in about 8 to 10 hours, so it was not surprising. It was after 3 am when I finally left the hospital. I went home and did a lot of praying. I did not ask for specifics. I handed you over to God and asked for acceptance, patience, and understanding. I told God to do whatever was in His plan for you, but to give me strength to accept it.

The third and fourth surgeries were the work of Dr. Remy Blanchaert, Oral Maxillofacial (OMF) Specialist. My left face had suffered a huge amount of destruction. Dr. Blanchaert had to repair full-thickness lacerations, a sizeable deficit caused by avulsed tissue, and a severed ear, that was displaced to the back of my head. He later told me that upon examination of the assorted facial fractures, he decided that they did not need adjustment. After careful debridement and suturing, there was still a hole to be dealt with. During the fourth surgery, a skin graft was applied. The skin was harvested from my left shoulder and attached to my face. After about two weeks, having failed, it was discarded. The hole healed under the care of Mike, as directed by Dr. Blanchaert. I am very grateful to the men I refer to as my face-savers.

I am resentful that my husband's family was not present for my loved ones during their extended nightmare and they have not shared their reasons for being neglectful. Loving support is so very important during traumatic times. It is a significant reason why I have made such a good recovery from serious injuries. I am saddened when I imagine what it must have been like for my family without loving support from all of the family.

(Eileen) When did you first hear that I had a brain injury?

(Mike) Probably not until several days later when you responded, according to hospital staff. I thought that you responded well to me but I would get reports that you were restless and could not follow commands. It was harder at first to think that brain injury was what it was because they had said that there was no cerebral hemorrhage.

During that critical first week, I was highly medicated with morphine. My family tells me that I seemed peaceful and my medical records reflect a GCS of six. I was in the process of fighting my way back to this world, however. According to my husband, one of my earliest achievements was the ability to stay awake for more than five minutes at a time.

(Mike) I had experience with people being A) knocked in the head and B) heavily drugged as you were. What they do at Shock Trauma is to keep you knocked out. By then your first surgeries were over and you were on a respirator in your room.

He told me of a stage when the nurses and therapists got me out of bed and made me stay in a chair, even though I cried and begged to get back in bed. Apparently, my internal clock had days and nights mixed up. During this time, when I was barely out of coma, they also had me out of bed, holding me steady on my feet to take a few steps. I thank God for determined, devoted nurses and therapists. Where would I be without them? However, my heart hurts for this woman. I still cry when I imagine her pain and misery. There were spoon feedings by my husband to avoid reinsertion of the feeding tube and everyone was constantly cueing me to keep me oriented to place and time.

(Mike) Then when the respirator was removed, you responded very childlike and confused. I did not think of it as a brain injury because my knowledge of it was less extensive than it is now. Like many people, when I thought about brain injury I thought about lack of mobility or a vegetative state - things like that. It was more of a confusion thing with you that was worse when I was not around. I gave a lot of credit for that to all the medication you were on.

My family has told me that I had wheelchair rides around the hospital. My daughter says that on one excursion to the main lobby of UMMC, I asked if I could sit in her lap. The staff kindly turned my bed around to give me a different view but when I was questioned about it later, I expressed disappointment. I wish I knew what was in my mind. When I earned a 3 to 5 on the Rancho Los Amigos Scale (Rancho Scale), I was transferred to Kernan Orthopaedics and Rehabilitation Hospital (Kernan) in Baltimore, Maryland.

> *(Mike) I do not think that it really hit me 100% that you had a brain injury, until they told me that they were transferring you to the TBI (Traumatic Brain Injury) unit at Kernan Hospital.*

In this stage, I was still highly confused and needed constant cueing to attend to any activity. My mind tended to wander and I was highly distractible. I will never have memory associated with this stage but my own medical records tell the story. I would have still been deep in my own world.

Rancho 3 to 5

The walk home from the park that day was filled with dread. I walked beside my older sister who was 7 or 8 years old. She was tenderly holding something against her forehead and the tracks of her recent tears showed on her grimy cheeks. What she was covering on her forehead terrified me. It was a fresh, brightly colored, swollen bruise, caused by me. I had killed my own sister! It did not occur to me to be comforted by the fact that we were walking home together. I just knew that it was the worst thing that I had ever done and that I should be punished.

The city of Montreal was a wonderful place in which to grow up in the mid 1950's. Although we were English, we lived in a French culture, which we absorbed in the best, most natural way. I felt both intimidated by and fascinated by the French and I did not understand why there were not more people like my family and me. We were three sisters, each 2 years apart, and I was in the middle. We would have been three, five and seven, or four, six and eight on that day. There was, of course, Mummy and Daddy, too. I did not like to get close to Daddy because I did not like him. He would say, "This is the smart one," with a sneer. Mummy cried a lot and never hugged me. She said, "I don't worry about you because you can take care of yourself." They were both very good-looking, and liked to party. My two sisters inherited the good looks; they were pretty girls and briefly enjoyed modeling careers. I was very different; I felt left out and tended to live in my imagination.

How we ended up at the park that day, I don't remember but all the fun-looking equipment excited me. The big sliding boards looked like mountains. What a breathtaking adventure it was to glide down from such a height. I felt like I was flying! I bet my wide-eyed look and big grin told the tale.

My happiness and excitement ended abruptly when I was coaxed into holding onto one end of what looked like a ladder balanced across a pole, with my older sister on the other end. I was first to be raised up in the air, dangling, while gripping one of the rungs. I was unnerved. Then, my sister jumped up, lowering me to the ground but I was too scrawny and dumb to hold her suspended. I did not want to go up again, so I let go of theladder. She fell and hit her head on one of the iron posts with a loud clang. Her wails of pain brought adults over to the scene. She explained the details of the accident between sobs and I knew that I was guilty of murder! I really was "an evil little bitch" like Mummy and Daddy always said. Our little sister appeared and we started on the long journey home.

I knew that I was going to get a beating, so I was rehearsing stories in my head. Our homecoming was eventful. My mother's hysteria, the crying and wailing of three of the females, my father's window shattering roar, and my stoic silence, while wetting my pants, was a scene worthy of broadcast. Daddy shook my skinny body, loudly demanding my reason for trying to kill my sister. I whispered my response, "I don't know." The beating that followed was for three reasons, first - attempted murder, second - stupidity and third - peeing in my pants again. Later, an unexpected visitor to our home, while passing by the open bedroom door, saw me lying on my bed, bruised and naked from the waist down. I just stared at the ceiling, too scared to disobey Daddy, who told me not to move.

Fast-forward 43 years to Shock Trauma in Baltimore, Maryland. My husband, children, and sisters were gathered at my side rejoicing because I was showing more signs of emerging from coma. In a baby voice, I asked my loving husband if he beat me because I was bad. I am shocked and distressed at my regression to my childhood. Worse than that, is the tremendous guilt I feel for the appalling insinuation of abuse by my heroic and loving husband. Mike barely held back the tears, while seething with hatred for the man really responsible for the abuse.

My actual return to consciousness happened about three weeks before memory returned. At first, there were just traces of memory, beginning two weeks post injury. First, I remember being roused by nurses telling me that I had to get ready for my appointment. Second, I remember being dressed in strange clothing. Last, I remember a very uncomfortable ride in the back of a van, strapped in a wheel chair. I am able to pinpoint the exact date of this memory from reading hospital records, and from my husband's testimony. Mike has told me that he arrived at Kernan just moments after my departure, having been delayed while shopping for new clothing for me. I also have a curiously funny memory of laughing like a TV character from the 70's, Arnold Horshack, from Welcome Back Kotter. The rough condition of my voice was a side effect of being recently extubated. My family remembers that voice very well from my days at Kernan.

The following is from my interview with Dr. Michael Makley, my neurologist, and the medical director of the brain injury unit at Kernan Hospital, where I had been his patient 5+ years earlier.

> What is your earliest memory of me? *Probably the most significant one was your facial injuries. Not only were you in an accident, but you also had a significant facial injury. I think that there were some fresh surgeries that were involved in your face, too.*

> What was your opinion of my brain injury? *I thought that it was a severe injury as I recall. You were not comatose, in a vegetative state. You were certainly very impaired.*

> Can you give me some specifics? *You were in a*

confusional state. You were having difficulty laying down new memory.

What were my major issues? *Your face and the skin grafts that had been done. The others were involved with your level of head injury; the inability to lay down new memory, and the inability to have any insight into your deficits. Actually, as I recall, those cleared quickly. You "came up" and began to work with the therapists.*

What do you remember about my family? *I remember your husband as being very supportive and always there.*

What would be your description of me at that time? *To be honest, the description I remember is probably angry. You were in a lot of pain and had a terribly disfigured face. The skin grafts were still so prominent, and they required a lot of care. Given those circumstances, I do not think anyone thought it was out of the ordinary. I think it is safe to say that you were somewhat angry when you were on the unit but you were not flat.*

Did I ask you many questions about my situation? *I do not remember many questions but there were comments about the circumstances. Someone had hit you, so it was such an unfair event that happened. Your husband asked many good questions about your outcome and such.*

Was I completely unaware? *Once you came up, I think you were aware of what happened to you but whether or not you understood the ramifications or had full insight I do not know.*

What concerns did you have when I was released? *Just that you would make it to your follow-up visits - maxillo-facial surgery and any orthopaedic surgery and that you get into your outpatient program.*

Were you concerned about my outcome? *I was confident that it would go well because you had done well here.*

What did you think/feel about seeing me here again as a volunteer? *It was good. I think that the Brain Injury Association of Maryland is a positive thing and I was glad to see you putting your energies toward that.*

How would you classify my recovery? *I would classify it as a very good recovery. Given your injury, I think that you are doing very well.*

What are some factors for a good recovery? *It's hard for me to say. I wish we knew. Certainly age. A younger age at the time of injury goes with a better recovery. I think that supportive families also go with a good recovery. I think that another thing that goes with a good recovery is pre-existing brain development. In other words, a more active or curious brain that is put to good use and has a lot of connectivity already developed generally does better than a brain that is less involved, less active and less curious about the world.*

Of what use could I be on the brain injury unit at this time? *Organizational stuff, like bedside functional evaluation forms, etc. Some people call it busy work but it helps keep the machinery of the business going. Another thing is reaching out to our patients and families and saying that I have had this experience, I've been here - that is invaluable. That is one of the great things about having BIAM right outside of our door - it is a good resource for our patients and families. So the role of patient educator or staff educator - to say what this person is going through.*

Dr. Makley kindly agreed to a taped interview and when I listened to it later, I was shocked at the sound of my own voice. I was much less fluent than I used to be.

Advocacy

There is an additional collection of memories in connection with a very important early function performed by Mike on my behalf - advocacy in the form of heated discussions with hospital staff. One memory is an argument I had with a nurse at Kernan who was trying to administer a medication, which had been discontinued. It was being administered by hypodermic in the abdomen (very painful.) She said that she would put in my record that I refused medication, which was inaccurate. Another was when I got into trouble for going to the bathroom by myself. I had called for help but eventually could not wait any longer. I was going to be assigned a sitter unnecessarily. Still another, which makes me wince, was the inappropriate application of ointment or cream to the hole in my face. Dr. Blanchaert was very angry. His instruction was saline-soaked gauze, only. When she rubbed the goop off my face, it felt like my skin was being peeled off. Each incident seems insignificant; but I want you to know that without the protection of advocacy, my situation would have been more fearful, lonely, depressing and frustrating, which would have interfered with my recovery.

Prayer + Faith = Miracles

Another kind of advocacy that was engaged in for me was prayer. To be able to lay a destructively stressful situation in the lap of one who is superior to all of us is comfort beyond imagining. When Mike was in danger of being overwhelmed by grief and anxiety, he handed over to God what was not his to control. In this way, he was able to survive what might have destroyed him. His nightly prayers to God, for strength to face what he had to, were answered. He was granted strength enough for all four of us. Two priests, who are also friends, visited the hospital when I was at my worst. Father Stan Janaites and Father Pat Tonry prayed over my helpless form. I was added to the prayerlist at St. Joseph's Catholic Community in Eldersburg, Maryland, and at my place of employment, there were prayer vigils. I am convinced that all of the positive energy that was sent to me aided in my return to life. My good recovery from serious injuries has nothing to do with luck but a lot to do with God's will.

When I lay helpless, between life and death, a note was left on my pillow - "Talitha koum." When Jesus first lived amongst us, he was something of a celebrity. Everywhere he went he was in great demand and although he must have been very tired at times, he never refused a request for help. On one such exhausting day, he had barely climbed out of the boat, having been across the lake preaching, healing, and performing miracles, when a synagogue official approached him named Jairus. The man's daughter was gravely ill and he begged Jesus to come to his house and heal her. A curious crowd gathered and followed. Within the crowd was a desperate woman, also very ill. She believed that if she could just get close enough to Jesus to touch his robe, then she would be cured. That is exactly what happened and when Jesus became aware of it, he let the woman know that she was cured by her own faith. Meanwhile, Jairus' daughter had died by the time Jesus and the crowd got to their destination. The family and servants were distraught and angry. "It's too late!" they said. Jesus calmly corrected them saying, "She's just asleep." When he was at the child's side, he took her hand and said, "Talitha koum," meaning, "Little girl I say to you, arise." She immediately came back to life to the great joy of her family. Mike left the note for me and I eventually opened my eyes. Was it a miracle or faith? Are they the same thing?

Emergence...

"Though I dream in vain, in my heart it will remain my
stardust melody, the memory of love's refrain."
-Nat King Cole

In the beginning there was emergence. My name for this stage should not be confused with the medical term which refers to the time when a patient leaves the state of deep coma and becomes more alert and responsive. I found descriptions of that part of my early recovery in my medical records but it will never be a part of my memory. I read about a confused, agitated, disoriented, and combative woman who could not focus on simple commands. The reading of these reported behaviors of mine is one of many sources of emotional trauma. I wanted to hold her, comfort her, and let her know that everything would be okay. She must have been so far away and scared...

Rancho 3 to 5

I explained the upcoming trip to the small occupants of the baby carriage. They listened with wide, unblinking eyes while I told of the adventure. It was a dream of mine to fly and I wanted to take my little companions with me. I had devised a foolproof plan that would enable us to soar away like the birds. I could not have said why I wanted to fly, only that I felt compelled to do it. I did not share my plan with anyone else because I did not want to run the risk of being stopped. The only souls of any importance to me were staring expectantly from the baby carriage. They belonged to me and I was taking them with me.

It was time, so I made my way to the bottom of the steps and looked up. It was a long flight but freedom was worth the effort. I gritted my teeth and started the difficult journey before my courage ran out. The baby carriage was heavier than I expected and I struggled breathlessly. I dragged us slowly up the flight of steps, holding the banister with one hand, gripping the carriage tightly with the other. I was afraid that the clattering noise might alert someone to my flight but no one appeared. I had to stop climbing every four or five steps to get my breath back.

I stopped at the top landing and looked back. It was such a long way down and I felt proud of my accomplishment. I followed the rail that outlined the small porch with my eyes, looking for the best spot. I positioned the carriage at the edge, under the rail and was relieved that it fit. I would not have been able to lift and hoist it over the top. With a mighty push, I sent the carriage over the edge and excitedly watched as my beloved baby dolls flew. I followed them down but I do not remember landing on the wood pile more than twenty feet below.

Reality

Back in the future was a memory of a soothing voice saying, "Your pain won't last forever. You'll be okay. Don't give up." It was probably my loving husband at this crucial time. I have just resumed this narrative, having taken a moment to dry my tears and calm myself. The memory of that voice is with me whenever I have an opportunity to comfort a survivor of brain injury or family member.

I am still deeply disturbed by imagined scenarios of what those days were like for me. I am haunted by images of possibilities which can turn into nightmares. I ceased reading my medical records during the first year of recovery. An understanding of the permanence of amnesia eventually settled in me so I abandoned the quest for recall, but not gracefully. My actual memories of the stage of emergence go in and out of focus like a camera recording the scenes. I was tender, uninformed, apathetic, untrained, and bewildered. I equate this stage with babyhood, complete with needed boundaries, within which I felt secure. My neurologist, Dr. Michael Makley, released me from Kernan, to the 24 hour care of my husband, Mike. His experience of over 30 years as a nurse prepared him in many ways but I think that there was no way for him to prepare to watch his wife struggle to recover from brain injury.

Eileen + Mike = Love

Mike cooked, did household chores, and helped me with personal care. He tenderly cleaned and dressed the still-open wound on my face, which helped it to heal better than expected. He at first escorted me on short walks around our yard for exercise. Later, I was able to stroll in the yard alone, closely watched through all the windows. I recall my excitement when Mike took me for my first walk outside our yard. My stamina at first was not sufficient for more than a very short excursion but I was happy to see the familiar sights of my neighborhood again. I required at least one midday nap at this time because my energy level dropped quickly.

The Thanksgiving holiday of 2000 was a collaborative effort by Mike and me to prepare the celebratory meal for our family. I directed the effort from a chair in the kitchen, struggling to remember details and to stay awake. My dear husband literally slaved over the hot stove, following my instructions. I proudly managed to bake Mike a birthday cake, however, to celebrate this additional important event which was on the same day. My own birthday had been celebrated at Kernan the month before but all I have in my memory is the flavor of coconut cake.

Disinhibition

My days were spent in my favorite chair, surrounded by books for reading and notebooks for writing. I did not answer the phone or the door and all arrangements for therapy and doctor's appointments were made by Mike. Occasionally, my apathy was shattered by irritation that I was not shy about revealing to anyone. Dr. Remy Blanchaert caught my wrath too many times. I would like to take a moment to talk about my relationship with Dr. Blanchaert. He was tall, dark, and handsome and in his mid-thirties at the time. When I knew him, I was growing through the developmental stages of childhood and adolescence. I was affected by his good looks, which made my behavior shy, awkward, petulant, and resentful. I was annoyingly outspoken and extremely sensitive at the same time. I felt humiliated to look at him because of my perceived resemblance to Quasimodo. I remember one incident when I was especially distraught about my ravaged face. I asked him if I would look like this forever. He explained to me that part of a good recovery was to have a positive attitude. I turned and looked at his handsome face and said loudly, "That's bullshit!" There was much laughter since several people were present. Dr. Blanchaert was understanding, patient, and caring. I will always be grateful.

This incident points out another aspect of my early recovery - disinhibition. According to my family, they were often treated to my new style of self-expression when visiting me at the hospital. Apparently I eventually ended up in a private room partly because of my sailor-like language. One incident still gives Mike and me much amusement. I was still wheelchair bound and waiting in line, somewhere at Kernan, to get my hair cut. I became irritated with a wheel chaired female in front of me and indicated my displeasure with my middle finger. Mike grabbed my hands, red-faced and laughing. Even Dr. Michael Makley was told quite strongly one morning in the hall outside my room that I would rather be glued to a tree than spend another day in his hospital. I was released the following day.

Mike did a lot of shopping for me when I was hospitalized. I needed comfortable, easy-care clothing when I was still relearning personal care and working on a daily regimen of rehabilitative therapies. He also helped me to use the washer and dryer at the hospital during his daily visits. Without him, I could not even find them. Although I remember very little of my time at Kernan, my husband is thoroughly satisfied with the therapy I received, even witnessing some of it. But my sisters, Lorinda and Debby, became emotionally distraught one day when witnessing my speech and cognitive therapy when I was still a 3 to 5 on the Rancho scale.

Their formerly very bright sister could no longer read or count.

When I could, I spent time at the small mirror in the bathroom of my last hospital room. The sight of my face and body was an unbelievable shock. Because I had no visual memory of the sight of these injuries when they were fresh and truly horrifying, the comments by visitors about how good I looked made no sense to me. What they considered to be vast improvement was total destruction to me. My brain had only recorded what I looked like before the motor vehicle collision. I was an average looking middle aged woman then but the current picture was grotesque. It was hard for me to celebrate with my loved ones and medical professionals how well I had recovered, when my last memory of me was of a healthful, uninjured, and unscarred person.

I also remember daily struggles with a CD player in my room which played my beloved Beatles if I pressed the right buttons. I wanted to hear the music constantly, but my own inability to remember how to operate the device left me frustrated and tearful. Occasionally, I would successfully figure it out and immediately drop onto a chair exhausted. The music touched me as never before. Paul McCartney's plaintive "Yesterday" left me sobbing forlornly on a chair by the window. There didn't seem to be enough tears to wash away the internal pain. I did not know it at the time, but labile emotions are common after brain injury. The music was provided by Mike and traveled with me from Shock Trauma to Kernan. I later learned that staff members at both hospitals have memories of Beatles music drifting out of my room. The music helped to keep me self-oriented.

What is vivid in my mind from those days is the view from
the window of the last room I had at Kernan. It looked out on an
expanse of lawn leading to the parking lot. I remember gazing
at the cars and people coming and going, looking for my family.
If I saw them coming, my excitement brought tears to my eyes.
Their arrival meant comfort and relief from my anxiety. My new
existence did not make sense to me and that scared me. There
was no logical progression of events in my memory leading to the
hospital. I had partial memory of a job waiting for me somewhere
and a feeling of something important left unfinished. I only
remember my last week at Kernan but family visits were the best
part. They made me feel loved and wanted. My beautiful Beth,
then 23, assumed the task of bathing her mother in the small
bathroom of my hospital room. She was so gentle and careful of
my many injuries. Her touch was comforting. Before long, I was
clean, powdered, dressed in a fresh nightgown, and tucked into
bed. My handsome son, Mike, then 27, discussed our favorite
subject with me - The Beatles. He was very interested in the
anthology I was struggling to read. I do not remember receiving
it, but it was a gift from my husband for my birthday, which I also
don't remember. My son tried to keep me oriented to place and
time by discussing the upcoming presidential election. Before they
left, they always made sure that I knew what day it was and where
I was and I tried very hard to remember for my next cognitive
therapy session.

While still at Kernan, I remember an irresistible impulse
to walk. This was an immediate reaction to getting rid of my

wheelchair. I made a willful and defiant decision one day to ride
the chair out of my room, and to walk back without it. I do not
remember where I left it, but the hospital staff questioned me about
its loss later. The refusal to have a wheelchair in my room gave me
a feeling of triumph. This simple act also made me feel powerful
and tall, even though I am actually short. The walls of the ortho/
rehab hospital were fitted with waist-high rails throughout. I
found this very convenient for my solitary excursions. Once I was
rid of the wheelchair, my hospital room was vacant in daylight. I
couldn't wait to be up and dressed. Like an obedient child, I made
my bed and tidied my room. I no longer took my meals in the
dining room, where I felt out of place. I was not comfortable with
all those strange people, and I was not interested in making friends.
I wanted to get away from there. At first I slid along the walls of
the TBI Unit, using the rails for support. It seemed to take hours
to make one round trip; the configuration of the hallways getting
me lost. I thought I counted hundreds of rooms. Memorizing the
numbers didn't help, because they would not stay in my brain very
long. I know now that there are 25 rooms on the unit, and my last
one was T904. My therapists managed to find me for the sessions; I
couldn't keep the times in my head.

Eventually, the confines of the unit were not enough to hold me.
If I saw an open door, I passed through it. My wanderings caused
some inconvenience for the hospital staff. When I wandered onto
a neighboring unit one day, a staff member took my wrist to read
the ID bracelet and referred to me as "Ms Cooper," questioning
me about my origin. The only legible name on the bracelet must
have been Dr. Carnell Cooper of Shock Trauma. I snatched my

arm away, and in a very haughty, childish voice declared that I had no idea who Ms Cooper was, and that I was leaving. I remember stalking away, but I don't remember where I went.

I think I remember my first outside excursion. It was during my last week as a patient. Mike was visiting and asked if I wanted to go outside. I excitedly grasped the opportunity, hoping that no one would try to stop us. That was the beginning of my hand-holding phase. I needed the security because I felt bewildered and scared everywhere. Mike helped me find clothing appropriate for the weather and led me outside. We headed for the old mansion, which was the original Kernan Hospital for Crippled Children. We did most of our sight seeing outside and I was especially fascinated with the old stables out back. The light quality, sights, sounds, and scents are still very strong and pleasurable. It was easy to imagine being cared for as a child in that beautiful mansion with acres of grass and giant trees for adventures.

Home

My homecoming was a blessed event. I was relieved to be in my home again, but all was not well. My troubled mind could not explain the vague, uneasy feelings. The spoiling of me by my husband started immediately, but I could not summon enthusiasm. I am certain that my manner reflected the distance I felt from life. There was a numbness that penetrated all the way to my soul; like viewing my life through a window.

Another purchase made especially for my homecoming was a new bed. Mike wanted to make certain that I had plenty of comfortable sleeping room because of my numerous injuries. My first night home, I slept in a new queen-size bed instead of the old full-size one. After being carefully bathed, I was neatly tucked in. One sleeve of my nightgown was slit to accommodate the cast on my left arm. As I drifted off to sleep, I felt warm, comfortable, and loved. I wanted desperately to remember what happened to me, but I was so tired.

First Sex

Shortly after the cast was removed from my arm, we engaged in our first sexual encounter. My assorted orthopaedic injuries had healed well. The hole in my face was closed and headaches from assorted skull fractures subsided. I could not explain why I felt so far removed from life but Mike was my anchor. I wanted to feel womanly and desired despite my scars and deformities. I think Mike was more scared than I was. He loved me a lot but did not want to hurt my still-tender body. We both worried needlessly; all was well. I felt like at least one part of my life was still normal and Mike's loving tenderness was a big part of it.

Reading and Scenarios

The activities of reading and writing filled my days. Reading was a slow and tedious process for me, however. I could read faster than one page per day by then, which was my speed while still hospitalized. But lack of comprehension, memory deficits, and other cognitive issues required that I reread the same pages several times. I tended to blame the author for my difficulties. At that time

I just figured that I was having a run of bad luck choosing books poorly written. I was not ready to believe that I had cognitive deficits. Books borrowed from the library were a heavy assortment for someone just a few months out of coma. The subjects were: brain function, the injured brain, personal stories about brain injury, and SAT tutorials (to prove to myself that there was nothing wrong with me.) The last selection is laughable now. Perhaps I was in denial. What do you think? One of the authors of a book about living with brain injury earned a very low level of my esteem. He theorized that someone with a brain injury similar to mine (moderate to severe) would be as good as he or she was going to be after one year. I was so mad, sad, and scared at the same time. I wonder if he ever actually knew anyone with a brain injury.

When I wasn't second guessing the credentialed and expert authors, I was busy with my own writing projects. The drive to record my thoughts of the time was irresistible. I wrote a series of essays about my experience as a patient, a trauma victim, and a survivor of brain injury. I called the short narratives "scenarios." I can't remember where I got the word but I liked the way it sounded. The following excerpt is from *Bad Day*. "I should have gone to therapy, but I could not face it. I believe that if I lie perfectly still until the pain subsides, then my skull won't fly apart...a tear escapes from my good eye and hit's the blanket...and I am angry because I am still alive." This is from *Madame Frankenstein*. "I am already tired of looking at my ruined body. My face frightens me the most...now I am monstrous." Just reading these narratives from the first six months post injury gives me the creeps. I was completely self-absorbed, depressed, and morbidly obsessed with anger and resentment. Still, I think that it is significant to note that I was capable of creative writing just three to five months out of coma! Also, as noted earlier, my sisters witnessed an *early* cognitive therapy session when I was still unable to read. I do not remember that time in my recovery, but I do remember reading The Beatles Anthology while still in a hospital bed! I remember struggling to read one full page in one day. The effort exhausted me. I think that these two facts of my recovery are remarkable. They point out my fierce determination to get better, and the accelerated speed of my recovery.

Exercise

The first year following the motor vehicle collision was extremely busy for me. I wanted to be "all better" as soon as possible. I attacked all my therapy sessions with the gusto of a resolute toddler. When therapy ended I launched myself energetically into exercising. I joined a local health club, and eventually became what my husband called a "gym rat." I started slowly, carefully following the exercise guide written for me by my physical therapist. Daily visits to the gym were very important to me, eventually similar to an addiction. Whenever my usual trip was not possible, my mood suffered. I could be morose and irritable, which could make everyone around me suffer. There was real stimulation for me when exercising and that just made me want to work harder. My workouts left me physically exhausted, serene, and relaxed, so I slept like a baby.

My first time swimming was terrifying. Certain that I would

drown because of not remembering how to time my breathing,
I did not want to put my head under the water. When I held my
breath successfully, I was so proud! The resumption of diving was
another feat for which I had to psych myself up. Although I dove
without difficulty (not expertly) pre-injury, I had developed a real
fear of forcefully entering the water head-first. With feet planted on
the cold concrete, my toes would creep to the edge and hangover
it and with arms similarly extended over my head, I tended to
stand like a statue. I wonder if my fellow swimmers noticed the
long hesitation. After a successful dive, I quickly fought my way
to the surface because I had become nervous about being deep
under water. Lap swimming required relearning a specialized
breathing technique. For someone who just a few months before
was intubated and on life support, breathe control was a challenge.
After about two years of practice, I was very much improved.

Neuropsychologists

Neuropsychological evaluations were also part of my early
recovery. A speech and cognitive therapist recommended it and
since I was still eagerly obedient, the appointment was made. Even
though the therapist explained what it was, I didn't get it. So I
went as a kindergartner on her first day of school. During the
psychological interview with Dr. Vince Culotta, and the subsequent
testing by assistants, I occasionally glimpsed some of my own
deficits, but I ignored them. When it was over, I was extremely
fatigued and experienced an uneasy foreboding. Some days
later, at the examination of the summary report, my reality was
presented to me. I experienced acute horror when informed that

I now resided in the world of brain injury and that there was no way out. What do you mean that there is no cure for brain injury? A good brain had been the one thing about me of which I was proud; now it was supposedly gone. The experience left me feeling depressed and inadequate -- like struggling through a tough test in school, then earning a failing grade. The neuropsychologist was a charming and kind man about fifteen years my junior, but I was so mad at him. I hope that Dr. Culotta can forgive me.

The second neuropsychological exam happened about four months later. You may wonder, as I do, what was the point? I think I was seeking a second opinion in order to disclaim the first. I was still telling myself that it was impossible for me to have a brain injury and not know it. Curiously, the second neuropsychologist, Dr. Mark Sementilli, reminded me of the first. My troubled brain wondered if there was only one type, and where do they come from? The second doctor administered the test himself, and his calm, quiet manner comforted me. I was determined to get a better grade this time, so I tried to stay focused. Since some of the same tasks were presented, I thought that it would be a piece of cake, like having the answers to the test ahead of time. I was dead wrong. The tension mounted as one task after another revealed deficits, even to me. The second summary report was an echo of the first. The existence of this unseen damage within my brain was real and there was minimal improvement in four months. "Oh, God!" I thought, "How could you do this to me?" Suddenly, the meaning of my existence was dark and cloudy. What I relied on lifelong, since my troubled childhood, was ruined. Scarlett O'Hara's plea at the end of Gone with the Wind was appropriate to me all of a sudden,

"Where shall I go? What shall I do?"

Counseling

My first choice was professional counseling. Why psycho-
therapy? I was following the very strong advice from the two
neuropsychologists. Suggested by one and confirmed by the other.
The commencement of talk therapy was just four months post
injury and continues. I had the extreme good fortune to find an
individual willing to devote as much time as needed to get me on
the right track. Dr. William Hopkins, Clinical Psychologist, is an
extremely patient, pleasant, and easy-going man who has chosen a
career perfectly suited to his personality. My memories of the first
weekly sessions are not sharp. What I remember is my impression
of the first office where we met. It seemed cavernous, with Dr.
Hopkins seated so far away from me. There was also a two-way
mirror on the wall of the office, fitted with shutters in the hallway. I
remember the day that I finally had the courage to ask Dr. Hopkins
who the individual was in the window. I explained that although I
was never able to catch the man looking our way, I was disturbed by
his presence. If Dr. Hopkins was surprised by my query, he didn't
show it. Instead, he clearly and patiently explained the image.
He even took me into the hallway to demonstrate how the set-up
worked. When he opened the shutters, the inside of his office was
visible. I was amused at my own mistake at having concluded
that the man in the window (mirror) was a stranger, instead of Dr.
Hopkins. Thereafter, I always checked that the shutters were closed
before entering his office – in case there were strangers lurking in
the hallway.

Everything scared me. I felt vulnerable and unsafe everywhere. I did not know it at the time, but I was suffering from post traumatic stress disorder. Dr. Hopkins did not rush me into revelations about myself. With his high intelligence and professionalism, he allowed me to take the lead. This method made me feel comfortable, instead of intimidated. Over a period of time, I was finally able to relax more in his presence.

Psycho-therapy offers a variety of uses for individuals with brain injury:

- A full-length mirror

    When we groom ourselves to start our day, don't we look for a mirror? Our personal steps of preparation may be many or few and a mirror is the guide. Your reflection is the conclusive evidence that you are complete and ready for the moment. As I have interacted with Dr. Hopkins over the past several years, he has reflected my behavior back to me, presenting a clearer picture of myself. Then I could choose to make adjustments as needed.

- A string for one's kite

    Settling into my new existence has been scary and even lonely because of a rootless sensation. I feel separated from myself and from life; amnesia is partly to blame. Conversations with Dr. Hopkins about myself past and present, the world around us, and even about the time of the trauma helps me to locate my spot. Once I know where I belong, I can maneuver myself into position and come in for a landing. Having some control over my life generates security.

- An alarm clock

Feeling isolated post-injury is very common. It is also easy to lose the ambition to be active in society again. Self-motivation is wonderful, provided you have some. When I ran out of it, motivation had to come from an external source. My main source was and still is my husband. Dr. Hopkins has been another source. He encouraged me to try different activities outside of myself. Becoming a volunteer with the Brain Injury Association of Maryland, writing this book, and going to college, are three of the suggestions. Becoming a part of society again has been a vitamin bolus for my ego, but I cannot take all of the credit. I thank God, my family, and Dr. Hopkins.

EMS Team visits

The heroic folks at Reese Volunteer Fire Company in Carroll County, Maryland were visited by me twice. The first time was about one week after my release from Kernan. My memory of that visit is vague but Mike tells me that it was highly emotional for everyone. The second visit was by invitation to their annual awards banquet. I was guest of honor and received warm applause, good wishes from everyone, and assorted gifts, which I treasure. Mike and I were asked to start off the dancing part of the evening to Gloria Gaynor's "I Will Survive." I also had the opportunity to speak in front of the group. During my thank you address, my husband tells me that everyone was in tears. I have a vivid memory of Sam Mann, EMS team captain, holding his dinner napkin to his face. There were car racing fans present, so I spoke of the recent death of Dale Earnhardt. He and I each sustained a basal skull fracture. I credited my survival to the dedication of the EMS team, who made a concerted effort to ensure that I did not lose respiration. According to comments made to me that evening, they were deeply touched by my speech.

Litigation

The motor vehicle collision that caused my injuries was not my fault. I had been a careful, deliberate, and focused driver with a clean record - never even pulled over by the police. The lesson here is that it doesn't only matter what kind of driver one is, serious injury can happen to anyone because there are other drivers on the road. When I was still in a coma at Shock Trauma, Mike found an attorney to deal with all the legal issues so that he could focus on his family.

The very skilled attorney, Michael Freedman, took my case. He apparently visited me in the hospital a couple of times and at home. I do not remember the visits. My first memory of Michael

Freedman was at his office in Owings Mills, Maryland. He was going over the accident report with Mike and me at a table. I was extremely dismayed to find out that a second driver, who also hit my car, had reported to the police that I had been weaving in and out of the left lane as he followed behind. He implied that the collision was my fault! I was incensed! How dare he describe my driving like I was drunk or careless? Michael assured us that this man would not be allowed to mess up the case. He was correct. I was so scared when we went to the courthouse one morning in May 2001. That was the date of the deposition. I didn't know what to expect, besides I had amnesia. What good was my testimony? The room, with one large table, was crowded with about ten people and the attorneys outnumbered the witnesses. We were there to give testimony under oath. Michael Freedman was intimidating and tenacious and I was glad that he was on my side.

By the time we finished more than three hours later, it had been established that driver #1, in a speeding pickup truck was distracted for a moment (reason unknown) and took his eyes off the road. When he looked again, my little car was in his path and it was over quickly. My car was struck head-on, overridden, and squished to the pavement like a bug. The collision happened entirely within a left-turn lane that I was in the habit of using as a short-cut to my home, ten minutes away. Driver #2, unable to avoid the accident also hit my car with his SUV. There was also a reasonable explanation offered for the so-called weaving. When trying to enter the left-turn lane, I probably saw the on-coming pickup truck and tried to get out of the lane. West-bound traffic to my right prevented my escape so I had to turn back into the lane and take the impact. Michael Freedman managed to make driver #2 look like a numbskull, as he stood over him during the cross examination. I was secretly cheering. When it was over, I encountered Driver #1 on the courthouse steps. He was a tall, lanky 28-year-old with a haunted look. I offered my hand to him and said, "I forgive you." He took my hand and mumbled, "I'm sorry."

He turned away with tears in his eyes but I knew that he felt better. At that moment I experienced a personal power that continues to inspire and comfort me – forgiveness.

On the way home, Michael Freedman told me that I had been an articulate and impressive witness in spite of the amnesia. The attorney for driver #1 later shared a similar opinion with Michael over the phone. The litigation was settled in my favor but that does not mean that I became rich as a result. The 28 year old driver of the pickup truck carried minimal insurance and had no assets. My medical insurance company at that time put a lien on the proceeds of the litigation. If my attorney had not negotiated successfully with them, they would have gotten everything. They settled for a smaller amount but I resented them for it. A portion of the income Mike and I earned paid their premiums for years. Besides, they don't have to go through life with a brain injury; I do.

Termination

During the first six months of my convalescence, I could not return to my job as a cost and inventory accountant. They required, however, periodic written statements from my primary care physician confirming my disability. Mike, bless him, took care of that business as well as everything else. One day I found the courage to answer the ringing phone, which was unusual for me. The woman who asked for me was from human resources at my place of employment. When she asked me how I was doing, I naively thought that she was genuinely concerned but that was just a shadow of things to come. I asked her to let my associates know that I appreciated all the cards and flowers and that I hoped to see them soon. She asked me when I would return to work full-time. I told her that I didn't know but that it was up to my doctor. I also asked her if she had been getting the physician reports. She said yes and then asked me to confirm the statement on the last report which said that I could not return to work at this time. When I did, she informed me that I was terminated. I became very upset and asked if my boss, the controller, authorized my termination and would she please have him call me. A letter of termination arrived in the mail the following week but I never heard from the controller. I still feel shaken by the encounter.

During outpatient therapy at Kernan, I was given a valuable leaflet from the Maryland Division of Rehabilitation Services (DORS) and one from the Motor Vehicle Administration (MVA). The first one was for occupational evaluation, training, and job placement. The second was for testing to be re-licensed after my neurological incident. The time spent at DORS yielded valuable information, but I was extremely lonely. I spent a week at their Workforce and Technology Center on Argonne Drive in Baltimore for vocational evaluation and it was the first time since being released from the hospital that I spent time alone in a strange place.

I came to the following important conclusions: A) I could never work at the same level again, and B) I was more vulnerable to stress and fatigue. I still sometimes grieve over conclusion A).

I managed to end my initial time with DORS on a happier note with the driving issue. An instructor came to my home to evaluate my knowledge, perception, reaction time, and other cognitive driving issues. Then, she took me for a test drive. My first time behind the wheel, post injury, was both terrifying and exhilarating. My protector and mentor (Mike) watched forlornly from a window as I backed out of the driveway. I did very well but the evaluator gave me some hints and clues to help me obtain my driver's license. I spent the next nine months submitting to numerous tests administered by the MVA, and I eventually acquired my learner's permit. But due to fear of failure, I waited the full six months before trying to get my license. During the time of my learner's permit, I could only drive when accompanied by my husband (or another licensed driver). I practiced very hard to stay focused and to pay attention to the other drivers. I no longer trusted them. Mike set up opportunities for me to practice parallel parking, using orange cones and broom sticks. Eventually, the time came for me to re-trace my drive home on that fateful day in October of the previous year. I drove all the way home from my former place of employment. I felt anxious and emotionally shaken, but determined. When *the* left-turn lane appeared, we were both disturbed to notice that the marks from the collision and the investigation were still visible one year later. When I was stopped in the lane, I needed my husband's help to judge a safe gap in the on-coming traffic because I was too shaken. That stretch of MD Route 140 had earned the nickname "suicide hill" because the downward slope was long and straight and motorists tended to speed. There are no jersey barriers separating the east-bound and west-bound traffic so "cross-over" is common and deadly. When I finally made the left turn successfully and started to follow the shortcut to my home, a small whimper of relief escaped from me. At the driving test, a very understanding examiner allowed me a second try at parallel parking when I messed up and even gave me some hints. My hands shook with excitement, and I skipped away from the car when I passed the test! A group of teenagers on the sidewalk awaiting their turns for testing congratulated me and we indulged in a joyful group hug.

911

On September 11, 2001, Mike and I were in Ocean City, Maryland. On that morning, I was watching live coverage of the twin towers in New York City on the television in our room while waiting to go to breakfast. I called to Mike to look at the TV because I didn't understand what I was seeing. Mike's shock and horror was reflected by everyone up and down the boardwalk in that resort town. Silent groups huddled in the doorways of storefronts to watch television. I thought that it was a strange sight to see all the tourists with their backs to the ocean. They were all appropriately grieving but I was numb. I felt far removed from everyone, like I was a different species. That was my first very strong perception of encapsulation. The feeling of a glass wall existing between myself and the rest of humanity continues.

Reflection...

"I'm a cork on the ocean, floating over the raging sea. How deep is the ocean? How deep is the ocean?"
-Brian Wilson

Emergence gradually transformed and became a stage I call reflection. Some of the aspects were curiosity, eagerness, anger, sadness, volatility, self-obsession, and yearning.

I had a voracious appetite for reading because my desire to understand myself was so intense. I couldn't relax for not knowing but knowledge requires understanding and reading comprehension was one of my significant deficits. It was a Catch 22 and it aggravated me. I was also disgusted with myself for being what I called a "retard." Now I know that abusing me because of my disability was as wrong as someone else doing it. I wish I had been kinder to myself. In addition, I was beyond the one year anniversary of my brain injury and according to some of the "expert" authors, as good as I was going to be. They will never know how desperately unhappy I was because of them.

Aside

If you are wondering where my father was at this time, he was relaxing at home about 50 miles away. However, he had remembered to call my sisters, who were visiting me one time at Kernan, to bring home pet food.

Depression

Emotionally, it was the best of times and the worst of times. On the good side, I was becoming more self-aware; on the bad side was self-disgust. Belief in the permanence of my injury was getting stronger all the time. Some of the information from all the books borrowed from the library was sinking in. I was noticing how my childish, sometimes outrageous behavior was affecting others. I worked hard on self-control but it was so challenging. Teaching me to step back and to take a breath was labor intensive. There was so much to remember in order to avoid over-reacting. I was always ashamed and felt like a failure when I threw a tantrum. Sometimes I cried so hard that my eyes felt like hot marbles. Growing up a second time is tough work. A sense that I was being punished for some unknown reason was so intense that I didn't believe in justice anymore. I was also in the midst of struggling with that terrible lost feeling. Like a cork on the merciless ocean, I had no direction. It seemed like there was no purpose in living. I longed to be normal, like everyone else, because I hated being different. I called my existence "exiled" because I was permanently separated from humanity. Even though I could touch others, including Mike, it seemed like everyone was speeding away from me and I was always trying to catch up. Cognitive deficits, including diminished comprehension, were to blame. Another reason for my sometimes bad behavior was depression. I felt soaked in it and I couldn't get rid of it. Whenever I was told how "lucky" I was, I wanted to spit. I hated being alive. I couldn't find anything to like about my new self. The ongoing struggle with depression seemed never-ending and I was so tired. It was like climbing a mountain after a prolonged illness. Sometimes I just wanted to disappear because I couldn't find the energy to continue the fight.

Facing every day with a brain injury can feel like the chains on Jacob Marley's ghost in <u>A Christmas Carol</u>. Frequent naps sometimes allowed me to escape, however, because in my dreams, I was smart, powerful, beautiful, and safe.

Counseling

Weekly counseling sessions continued with Dr. Hopkins. It was not easy, at first, to open up to Bill, especially about all the ugliness inside me. Very patiently he waited months for me to break out of my "best behavior" façade. Sometimes I was angry, over-emotional, and unreasonable. At other times, I was silently brooding and morose. Occasionally I was bright and sunny, like a chirping sparrow. I will admit to you, reader, that I was not always honest with Dr. Hopkins about how I felt or about my deficits. I did not tell him that I wished I was dead, either. Do you think that he was fooled? Unlikely - he's way too smart. Some of you may wonder about talk therapy and how it works. In my opinion, the most important element for successful counseling of this kind is trust. The establishment of a trust relationship on both sides is essential. Another very important factor is comfort. Talking should be effortless, like spending time with a good friend or neighbor. I will tell you that at that stage of my recovery I was still deeply withdrawn so our relationship took many months to develop. I am very grateful to Dr. Hopkins for having the patience to wait for me to catch up.

Disinhibition

The self-confidence I once relied on was wiped away by the injury and self-control was replaced with disinhibition. The inability to self-censor is a common side-effect of brain injury and should not be confused with non-inhibition, which is the lack of self-imposed suppression that we learn as we mature. Dr. Hopkins was witness to more than one instance of my disinhibition. During some early visits, my insurance company was extraordinarily tardy with coverage. When speaking to a clerk at the insurance company from Dr. Hopkins office, for about the tenth time on the same subject, I became impatient and said, "Which one of us has the brain injury? I keep forgetting." I haven't trusted myself to behave publicly as well as I used to so I have felt more anxious about being social. Eventually Bill (Dr. Hopkins) told me that I was *more* disinhibited when he first met me. That makes me cringe because I know that, even recently, I have blurted out ugly words or phrases. He has never shown shock or dismay when I have misbehaved but his gentle chiding or raised eyebrow have made me feel ashamed. Self-confidence was a hard thing to lose, once possessed. Dr. Hopkins is Bill to me because I am most comfortable with him on a first-name basis; it is not due to lack of respect.

Defiance

The "very short hair" phase was also at this time. It lasted for over two years. The first relieving hair cut at Kernan was the catalyst. My head was partly shaved on one side and my medium length hair was left on the other. The longer hair was matted with blood and surgical debris so I felt so much better when it was all gone. I have concluded that I had two main reasons for keeping my hair very short. A. I was still awkward with personal care, so it was just easier, and B. I emerged from the tunnel as a different person, so I was being defiant about it.

Menopause came next. Thankfully, it was an adventure that I don't have to repeat. I was having a tough time coping with all the damage to my brain, face, and body. Having to face aging in addition, represented by menopause, was just too much. My gynecologist seemed bored with me, since I was not making babies. I had many concerns but he wouldn't even return my phone calls, so I dropped him. My next gynecologist was a female and a pleasant change. She examined me with gentleness and even showed concern about the recent trauma. I tried two different kinds of hormone replacement therapy for almost a year. In the end, I couldn't stand the side effects and I was terrified of breast cancer so I stopped. After the brain injury, it seemed like my system was extra sensitive to medication. Unfortunately, this very nice doctor left the practice. My next gynecologist was a small, Asian woman who recommended a natural substance, black cohosh, as a substitute for HRT. Black Cohosh gave me mild relief from my symptoms but after about a year I discontinued. I was not symptom free but I didn't want to take medication for it. Sometimes I suspect that my continuous overheated condition is also due to brain injury. In a few years, I would be certain.

Self-consciousness and Insensitivity

When one becomes older, there is a natural expectation of a more relaxed temperament and more wisdom. I was no different. As a youth, I pictured my mature years as a time of less intensity. I assumed that my physical appearance, social acceptance, and sexual fulfillment would no longer take precedent over everything else. I was wrong.

My one-sided facial paralysis and scarring made me want to turn away from everyone. At first, I didn't want to show my face to anyone. Going out in public could not be avoided but I was painfully aware of every glance or stare.

There was an incident at a radiology waiting room that still makes me uncomfortable. I was quietly reading a magazine when I became aware that the woman to my left had been openly staring at my face. She looked away when I glanced in her direction but I caught her sneaking another peak when my turn was called.

A couple of incidents in the locker room of the gym where I had membership were also very awkward. While dressing after my shower, I noticed a child staring and pointing at my midsection (the scar from the laparotomy was still vivid.) His mother covered his eyes and jerked him away, making me feel like a monster. On another day in the locker room I bumped into a woman I had not seen since the accident. When she saw me, she drew in her breath and in a shocked voice asked what I had done to my face. Was I in a fire? She asked.

Another individual at the office where I volunteered asked if the mark on my face washes off. I am sure that she did not mean to be cruel. Nevertheless, I felt very uncomfortable. In addition, when I was present a vendor selling his product was entertaining the office staff with descriptions of brain injured folks he had met. He pulled his lip down on one side to further mimic and imply mental retardation. I was shocked but not sure how to react so I did nothing.

One day, when walking in my neighborhood, I stopped to talk with a woman I have known for thirty years. She kindly asked how my recovery was going. Unfortunately, she ended our conversation with an attempt at humor. She said that the children in the neighborhood who used to call me "the walking lady" could now call me "the scarred lady."

Another instance was a business meeting with an office manager. I was attempting to get a clear explanation of a convoluted statement of account. After several minutes of my repeated and unanswered questions, she and her associate showed clear exasperation and impatience. They stated that they had worked on the statement for a long time and it was quite clear, so why didn't I understand? Thereafter, one of the women treated me very coldly whenever we met. A spokesperson, in their defense, said that they were not used to "dealing" with a person with a brain injury. To me this was a confirmation of my exile from "normal" people.

Still, another time I listened as a woman suggested that the brain injured crew of volunteer workers is given very simple tasks because otherwise, they might wander around and get in the way. I was angry but I spoke evenly and specifically in our defense. Why is it hard to understand that most of us are capable and productive individuals? If I was thoughtless and uncaring of persons with brain injury before I was injured, I am ashamed.

Libido

Intense sexual desire can be wonderful and terrible at the same time. My libido had not only reawakened, but sex filled my thoughts more than I ever remembered. I had not felt so sexually stimulated since I was a virgin. Way back then I tended to blame it on the advent of the Beatles, when my hormones were newly released and raging. Later, it was because I had fallen in love with Mike. Speaking of whom - he was thoroughly delighted with this new aspect of my personality. He wondered, rightfully, where this engaging eroticism had been. The change in me heated up the sexual side of our marriage to a degree perhaps not intended for 50-somethings. My husband told me that being with me was like being with a sixteen year old, which was a little scary. My heightened libido did occasionally cause too much stress and pressure. I didn't know the mechanism of the brain injury that caused this phenomenon. My feelings alternated between delightful enjoyment and fear of becoming a "dirty old broad" chasing after men in my wheelchair at the retirement home. Since I was somewhere in the midst of the second maturation process in my life, developmentally I may well have been a teenager. Body-obsession was present and full-blown. I became reacquainted with pleasuring me, which was retro-activity from when I was an adolescent. I needed to relieve the constant tension I felt.

Humor

According to my husband, this phase of my maturation contained adolescent-like moments. For instance, on a trip to McDougalls Drug Store in Eldersburg, Maryland, our home town, laughter got the best of both of us. While Mike waited at the counter to make his purchase and to drop off a prescription, I entertained myself by reading product labels. McDougalls is a small pharmacy that carries some "old-fashioned" and rare home remedies. I was delighted to come across two products on the same shelf with intriguing names - Crack Cream and Butt Paste. I was still working on self-control so in one fervent moment, I blurted out the first word of the second product, remembering to slap both hands over my mouth in order to stifle the second word. As the echo of that one word (butt) traveled around the small space, Mike's startled reaction at the counter initiated my giggling. He quickly gathered his purchases, rescued me from the embarrassing scene, and herded us through the store with surprising dignity. As soon as we reached the parking lot, we collapsed into helpless laughter.

On another outing, we were enjoying a delicious dinner at a restaurant. In the middle of our conversation, I startled Mike, myself, and everyone present with a sudden, loud burp. For a moment, we were speechless with shock and then the laughter started. While I hid behind a cloth napkin, Mike teased me about not being able to take me anywhere. The contrast between the formerly self-controlled and well-behaved woman and the somewhat disinhibited version of me is still amusing. These two funny stories illustrate that recovery from brain injury is not all long faces and sadness.

Surgery

During reflection time, which coincided with self-imposed isolation, I seemed to become increasingly vain. Please be aware, reader, that I was never a beauty, even as a child. But suddenly, my appearance was of great interest to me. I blame it on the scars and deformities of which I was intensely self-conscious. Severe, soft-tissue damage and facial fractures had changed my appearance in subtle ways but noticeable and unwelcome to me. The healed facial fracture where my jaw attaches to my upper face has a visible and tangible lump under the skin. I hate the feeling of it when applying moisturizer. My upper, left face is paralyzed; my right ear is significantly lower than my left. I have a long, curved scar emerging from my hair at my left temple area, running down my face, under my chin, and a little down my neck. My left eyelid droops slightly; my whole face is tilted on its axis to the right, and I have some permanent hair loss on the left side only. My head is so full of scars that I have an extensive collection of cow-licks and natural parts in my hair. My body has a list of scars and deformities that I will discuss later.

Dr. Remy Blanchaert performed three surgeries on my face, stabilizing it and laying a good foundation for the next step - plastic surgery. Dr. Navin Singh, plastic and reconstructive surgeon, has made a series of subtle changes to my face, greatly improving my appearance and I am very grateful. He has expressed to me on numerous occasions that he cannot erase the ravages of time and trauma but he can de-emphasize scars and deformities. He has kept his word.

By the time the third anniversary of the motor vehicle collision came and went, I had faced eleven surgeries. During my emergence and reflection stages I was either recovering from or planning my next surgery. Since my injured brain is more sensitive to medication and my emotional state is more delicate, each instance at the hospital was fresh trauma for me. I was very grateful for my husband's support and advocacy. I must have been a very challenging patient.

Not all the surgeries were planned, however. An extraordinary thing occurred more than once and it was frightening at the time. When my car was demolished around me, apparently, pieces of the windshield managed to enter my body through open wounds. Some of the foreign objects worked their way to the surface and came out of my skin of their own accord. On these occasions, I would hear the tell-tale plinking of a shard of glass hitting the floor when I undressed. At other times, the glass would get stuck in my skin on the way out and required a doctor's help to finish the job.

One of my orthopaedic surgeons, Dr. Andy Eglseder who repaired my badly damaged left arm beautifully, also removed some glass protruding from my arm at a follow-up appointment in his office. On another occasion, there was a sudden onset of severe swelling and discomfort in my left arm, which had me back at Shock Trauma. That emergency surgery terrified me; I was scared of amputation. When I woke up, my arm was still in place and was also relieved of the discomfort of foreign objects.

The last episode of foreign objects in my arm and upper chest was assigned to Dr. Navin Singh. That was our first meeting. On the morning when I reported to the hospital for surgery and was being prepped, I asked Dr. Singh about the awful-looking scar down the center of my body. Can he improve it? What followed was my first experience with an extraordinarily embarrassing evaluation by a plastic surgeon. In the presence of my husband and another nurse, Dr. Singh's assistant, and with the exam room door opening and closing, I was suddenly standing naked before everyone. I could hardly speak from the shock. That surgery was successful thankfully and the last of the foreign objects was removed.

On another ride to the hospital for more surgery, I was trying to appreciate the beautiful sunrise through the windshield. It was quiet in the car except for the music on the radio. An old song from the sixties, How Can I Be Sure? by the Rascals, was playing. I have always loved the waltz tempo of this one, and imagined myself skimming lightly over ice, perhaps with a graceful spin. Ice skating can feel like flying. The song is about love's uncertainty but a glance at the man behind the wheel was reassuring. He gave me a smile and patted my hand. Then my thoughts turned to the loving letter he wrote and gave me the night before. Read it for yourself and tell me what you think.

Eileen -

Do not be afraid. God is with you. That is the most important thing to remember. Of much less importance is, I am with you, too. I will be here with you as long as you live. And if God lets me, I will look after you after my life is over.

Do not be concerned about obtaining or retaining worldly knowledge. God has given you a high I.Q. and He will work through you and the gifts he has given you. Accept Him as a child accepts Love.

Do not rehearse what you want to say. Think about it. Then pray to the Holy Spirit and He will give you the right words to say. You will be amazed at how easy it is.

Do not try to change who you are right now. You are the person you are by going through all of these experiences. You were meant to go through all of your yesterdays, both good and bad, to become who you are today. And again tomorrow, and again the next day.

Do not say, "I knew so much then" or "I contributed more then" or "I liked the way I looked then," because "then" you knew nothing about today's joy and love. Because "then" you hadn't yet contributed to the complete happiness you have given me, your children, the medical people, and all of us who have witnessed the miracle of your return to life. And "then" you didn't have the wonderful look you have now. The look of someone who was told "You still have a lot of work to do;" the look of someone who was comforted by the voice of the Lord.

We have all been given gifts. All the Docs who took care of you, to all the Sam Manns who cry at the sight of your recovery, to the baby we hear crying in the grocery store. We have been given the free will to decide to use those gifts.

As we run the race and take the journey, we touch and influence so many people without even knowing it. That is how our spirit lives on. If we live to be a hundred or only for a few days, we are not wasted. We have done what we were sent to do. We have free will. It is not easy. We forget and slip. But as much as we love and forgive those we love with all of our imperfections, imagine the great love God has for us.

If you are still confused about how you feel about your surgery, before you go to sleep ask God to send the Spirit to you and you will awake with the right decision. Then whatever it is, stick to it.

Accept that some of the Docs who were so very important in touching this critical time of your life must move on as instruments of God to touch other people's lives. Believe me;you touched their lives, too. As John Lennon touched your life, all the devoted fans touched the lives of the Beatles, too and made their lives good.

It is all so immense; we couldn't try to even comprehend how all of us touch each other in God's plan. So don't try to understand. Don't strive for

*knowledge. It will come by itself. Instead, pray to
accept as a child accepts.*

*Heaven is having the peace of seeing and feeling the
love of God. Hell is seeing it, then ceasing to exist and
never feeling it.*

I have told you all I know. I love you.

*Love,
Michael*

I awoke in the morning certain that I had made the right
decision so then I had to face and cope with all the discomfort for
me and for my family. Since the trauma I have had many surgeries
but this one was different. I had elected to have cosmetic surgery
on my face and body to minimize scarring and deformities. I was
in the care of the extraordinarily gifted Dr. Navin Singh. He had
told me that the surgery would be more than six hours long. I was
terrified. After many surgeries, I was still not accustomed to it.
Each time yielded fresh trauma. I was also unhappy to add more
amnesia to my collection.

At the hospital I had to endure what seemed like "public
nudity." I felt like all of Baltimore had seen me naked. I had to
stand patiently while my face and body was examined, poked, and
drawn on. My audience was very attentive but I gazed at the ceiling
trying to forget that I was naked. My wrist still hurt where the I.V.
line was inserted. Why did they always say that it only hurts for
a moment? When it was time to say goodbye to Mike, I almost

chickened out. I must have been crazy to put him and me through more traumas. He would have to wait somewhere scared for several hours while God knows what would be happening to me.

The wheel chaired ride to the surgical suite went too fast. In what seemed like seconds, I was lying on a table, told to relax and breathe deeply. Tears of terror rolled out of the corners of my eyes. Didn't they know? Couldn't they see? Then I thought about what Mike wrote and I remembered that God was with me, even in the O.R. The strange, metallic taste in my mouth was my last memory.

My next memory was asking the man caring for me in another room, "what time is it?" Upon hearing the answer, I realized that I had lost another six hours to amnesia. I felt cold and thirsty, my throat hurt, and I needed my lip balm. To my joy, Mike appeared and all was well. The cup of hospital tea that he helped me drink tasted like the best I'd ever had. When I was transferred to my room, I had to endure the usual nausea and vomiting. Why can't they ever prevent it? I felt like I was hit by a truck again and so very grateful for pain medication. After two lonely and boring nights in the hospital, I was released and anxious to get home. Mike told me that I dozed off and on in the car all the way home.

To say that I was uncomfortable is not nearly descriptive enough. Staples and stitches in my scalp, on my face, and on my abdomen made me squirm. I was also dismayed to carry around a pair of drains attached to my middle. I had to pin them to my clothing. The act of emptying the collection bulbs caused a sucking sensation deep inside my body and I retched. The extreme discomforts only lasted about three weeks. Soon, I not only felt good but I was beginning to see my improved appearance through the swelling and bruising. Mike, of course, had been with me through it all. As my flesh began to recover from all the surgeries, I was more gratified with the results and I began to feel more confident in public. I sometimes thought of Dr. Singh as a psychologist with a scalpel.

Amnesia

Amnesia was and still is an important factor in my depression, misbehavior, and lost feeling. At first, the effect was not clear to me. Months passed before I realized that I was so very uncomfortable whenever I heard my lost time mentioned because I don't remember it. It seemed unreal. I had no idea what I did, who I knew, how I behaved, or how I felt. I understand now that the time spent reading my medical record was a pitiful effort to restore my memory. For a while I didn't understand about the permanence of amnesia. I assumed that in time I would remember everything. I even started believing that some of what I imagined was actual memory.

Throughout the period of reflection I was still anguished due to lack of memory. I thought that I had discovered a really good idea to help fill in the holes - photographs of me during *the big blank*. Back in emergence stage, when I visited Reese Fire Company, I was shown the photographic records of the rescue. I badly wanted to look at them over and over again. They were undeniable evidence that the incident actually happened. My friends at the fire station responded with understanding and the photographs arrived soon. My emotional response was overwhelming. As I gazed at my familiar but lost red car, I believed that my rescue was miraculous. Members of the EMS team were gathered around my demolished vehicle, obviously hard at work to pry it open. The other photographs depicted - first an empty gurney - then a full one, cargo unknown, because the patient's privacy is protected. Another photograph records them loading me into the ambulance. The waiting helicopter was about one mile away from the site. I tried to memorize the look of the whole scene. The gathered witnesses - the looks on their faces - the number of rescue vehicles - the distant white pickup truck - the black SUV on the rear driver's side of my little red car - the familiar road signs - all this was deeply meaningful to me. It was a beginning but I wanted more.

Next, I turned to Shock Trauma because I knew that a patient's case was sometimes documented with pictures. I hoped that I had been one of those patients. I was wrong and deeply disappointed. I never obtained a photograph from them, and I don't even know if they exist. As a survivor, I would like to make a very strong suggestion to Shock Trauma to photograph *all* unconscious patients and to make the pictures available, in addition to the hospital records. There may be other deeply frustrated former patients like me.

When I was with the OMF team of University of Maryland Medical System (UMMS), I remember posing for pictures at different stages of my treatment. I wanted very much to see what I could not remember. Dr. Remy Blanchaert responded to my request with one graphic and startling digital picture - a head and shoulders shot. I was unconscious, a breathing tube protruded from my mouth, and my face and neck were badly swollen. My left face had a huge, open wound where the flesh had been torn away and my left ear had been displaced toward the back of my head. Half of my head was shaved and I was so lacerated and swollen, that I was unrecognizable. I have just dug this picture out of the box of hospital records to view it again. It is still a shattering experience but part of my reality. When I was given this graphic picture, I was not appropriately responsive due to my brain injury. Based on his dismayed reaction, Dr. Blanchaert may have thought that he caused more psychological damage. He wouldn't give me any more pictures and he has since moved to Kansas. I have not seen him in several years but if

I could get a message to him now, I would say, "Thank you for saving my face Dr. Blanchaert and thank you for caring about me. You didn't hurt me and I am better for knowing you."

My small collection of pictures has filled some holes and I am grateful to have a little something to help me feel more connected to that woman in transition. I would say to anyone with a loved one in a similar situation, "Please journalize, document, and photograph your loved one's time in *the big blank*. Some day you may be able to satisfy his or her intense curiosity."

Social Security

The two-year struggle with Social Security finally came to an end and I felt like the winner of a tug-o-war contest; we both got dirty. Convincing the bureaucrats that brain injury is a real disability was frustrating, humiliating, and discouraging. Just having to talk to them frequently ended with my emotional breakdown. I was fighting for my livelihood and they treated me like a pesky mosquito. One clerk asked me if there was a McDonald's in my neighborhood. When I answered yes, she suggested that I apply for work there, since it should be easy to run a cash register with my accounting background. A highly emotional, out-of-control scene followed, from which my husband had to rescue me. I don't know if I will ever understand why the reams of documentation I submitted were not good enough. Coincidently, when I enlisted the help of a group of disability experts, the battle ended suddenly and in my favor.

Scenarios

The many personal accounts and books about brain injury I read inspired me to submit my work to assorted magazines. I rewrote and combined some early "scenarios" for a finished product that I bundled and mailed, along with a cover letter, to about six periodicals. I only received one answer, which was a rejection, and I was deeply hurt. Any other reaction was precluded due to my self-obsession and hyper-sensitivity. In my injured world, this was evidence that no one cared about brain injury and I concluded that what I had left, intellectually, wasn't of any value. I also thought that if I could not reach anyone with my writing, there was no way out of my isolation. Another serious bout with depression had commenced.

Exercise

Another weapon against depression was physical activity. I had a very strong dedication to my exercise routine at the gym. I could leave the world of deficits and disability for a while and spend time in a world of pleasing body sensations. Feeling my body strengthen and experiencing the tranquility of endorphins was a treat I didn't like to miss. My exercise routine also included lap swimming. The smooth, buoyant movement of my body through the water and the focus on counting and breathing, made this exercise almost hypnotic. My best sleep was after swimming.

When I wasn't at the gym, I was walking. Sometimes I was able to walk off an emotional upset and return home much calmer. One of my neighbors said that she lost count of the number of times I passed her house. The rhythmic movement of my body at my will gave me a feeling of control that had been missing for a while and I loved it. Sometimes I wished for more hours in the day so that I could walk more. On days when I felt the worst emotionally, I was tempted to walk all the way to Westminster, a small city ten miles from my home.

Volunteerism

An occupational therapist at Kernan gave me a brochure for DORS, and while at DORS, I was given a copy of the Maryland Directory of Brain Injury Resources, published by the Brain Injury Association of Maryland. My counselor, Barbara Krupnik, thought that I might be able to find a useful resource. She was correct.

I had gradually become aware of a peculiar restlessness and I was no longer apathetic and bewildered. A small income from Social Security Disability (SSDI) was finally a reality so there was more financial stability. Physically, I was much stronger due to all the exercise. Since ten of the eleven surgeries were over, I felt a little less self-conscious about my appearance.

The resource directory was my constant companion. I spent hours going through it, hoping that an idea would occur to me. It seemed like I had been standing still forever and I longed to be interactive again in the community. An entry near the beginning of the directory drew me:

> Brain Injury Association of Maryland, Inc.
> 2200 Kernan Drive
> Baltimore, MD 21207
> Phone: (410) 448-2924
> Toll Free: (800) 221-6443
> Website: www.biamd.org

I returned to this entry frequently, wondering if this was it. My husband explained to me that the address was Kernan Hospital. With encouragement from Mike and Dr. Hopkins, I found the courage to call and ask about volunteer work. I spoke to a very nice woman named Suzanne Kantt, Assistant Director. She invited me to attend an informal meeting about volunteering. I took her advice and I was captured. After a pleasant interview with Diane Triplett, Executive Director, during which I apparently displayed my high anxiety, an odyssey of pleasure, education, and fulfillment began.

Exploration...

"Help me if you can. I'm feeling down, and I do appreciate you're being 'round. Help me get my feet back on the ground. Won't you please, please help me?"
-The Beatles

I was thus launched into exploration. I landed in a world that I thought was lost to me forever.

Years ago, when I became an accountant, I thought that I had found a perfect match for my strengths and talents. I was precision and detail oriented. I could sort through a tall, messy stack of paperwork and computer printouts littering my desk and convert it into a neat, thorough, and informative report to present at a finance meeting in the morning. I worked long hours into the evening and on weekends. My life revolved around spreadsheets, account analysis, journal entries, production costs, and inventory levels. I was sharp -- determined to learn anything anyone cared to teach me. My bosses marveled at the quality and quantity of work I produced. That woman was lost in a car wreck in October 2000.

I emerged from the coma in pieces, like a scattered jigsaw puzzle. After six years, I was still working on the puzzle, realizing that some of the pieces were missing. I suspect that this work-in-progress will be very different from the original, when I am a finished product. Any cost and inventory accountant in manufacturing is familiar with the phrases used in the previous sentence. I am highly amused to describe myself in the same way as I once discussed apparel production.

I also suspect that this stage of exploration is current and ongoing. Why? Because I cannot see the end, as I can with all the previous stages of recovery. Daily, I experience some of the following: excitement, education, inspiration, exhaustion, anxiety, frustration, and therapy. My days are full of exercise for my brain and body, volunteering in the brain injury community, and family enjoyment.

Stepping away from self-imposed isolation was terrifying, and I needed my husband's strong support to do it. I was not happy when I was avoiding the world, but my anxiety level is much higher now. Manifestations of my brain injury are fully exposed to public scrutiny. When I become aware that some of my deficits are revealed, I feel humiliated and defiant at the same time. I sometimes wonder if my extreme self-consciousness about my cognitive abilities is entirely under my control. Whatever happened to the strong, self-confident woman who could rise up at high-level meetings, holding her own and scared of nothing? My desire to learn more about this new world in which I exist, however, is much stronger than my anxiety. So I continue, but sometimes I am completely exhausted. I no longer require a midday nap, but I am usually in bed early, sometimes by 9 pm.

On a typical day, you may engage in multi-tasking, problem solving, prioritizing a long list of tasks, and retiring at the end of the day, tired, but satisfied with your accomplishments. You even find the energy, somehow, to repeat it after a short rest. For a brain injury survivor to face such a day, occasionally, is manageable; to try to do it several days in a row may yield dramatic results. Dizziness, slurred speech, marked clumsiness, lower level cognitive abilities, crankiness or over-emotion are just some of the possibilities. I sometimes need a few days to recover from such exhaustion. I can only complete a much smaller list of tasks than I used to, and I am not always content about it. My more frequent errors are even harder to accept.

The paragraph above answers questions frequently asked of me. Why are you disabled just because you have a brain injury? Why can you not be an accountant anymore? Can't you still do math, or use a calculator?

Volunteerism

I started my volunteer career with the Brain Injury Association of Maryland on June 1, 2003. I felt like a little rabbit in a big, open field, outside of her warren. I have not been so scared since my first day of school. I was embarrassed to expose all of my weaknesses in public, and I longed for the strength and self-confidence of my former self.

My boss, Diane Triplett, is the executive director. On my first day, she outlined the association's needs and her expectations. Even now, I remember with gratefulness, her kindness, and understanding. The association needed help administratively - everything, from filing, bulk mailing, and photocopying, to projects that are more complex. In a comforting way, Diane expressed that she was not as concerned with errors as I had experienced in my pre-injury career. She made it clear that the association has significant understanding of persons with brain injury, and would benefit from any help I could offer.

As I listened to an outline of the tasks available, I was intrigued by one and terrified by another. Working on the newsletter, <u>Head Stand</u>, attracted me. I love to write. However, the thought of taking or initiating telephone calls gave me a headache. How could I help someone else when I could not help myself? Many months later, Diane expressed to me that my high anxiety was evident. I must have been delusional, because I thought that I was completely under control, and that everything was hidden.

The assistant director, Suzanne Kantt, patiently shared her great knowledge with me. What a good teacher she was! My self-confidence soared when she was present. In the beginning, Suzanne showed me very simple tasks, and as my skills expanded, so did my independence. I like to think that I had graduated from one who was aided, to an aide.

I remember, with amusement, my first attempt to go to the mailroom alone. Kernan Hospital is a 150-year-old facility with two or three additions on different levels. I journeyed from one building to the next successfully, using the route that Suzanne showed me. My first wrong move was going through a door in the stairwell to the left, instead of to the right. I ended up in a place that I have not found since. A kind staff member found me lost and wandering. She guided me back to the stairwell and pointed out my error. Even now, I feel like I spent time behind the looking glass.

At first, I worked alongside an extraordinarily patient woman named Barbara Sembly. She was the administrative expert. I benefited greatly from her instructions and her knowledge of the office layout. The greatest thing that she did for me was when she allowed me to sit by her side as she worked. I observed what she did, how she did it, and most importantly, her gentle, unhurried manner. I still have not mastered the last one. Barbara Sembly reminds me of Dr. Hopkins - calm, even-tempered, unruffled, and easy to be with. They are both very good role models.

My first successful telephone experience at BIAM occurred as I sat shoulder to shoulder with Barbara. With a twinkle in her eye, she encouraged me to answer the phone when it rang. As I handled the call, Barbara stayed close to me with smiling support, and when I hung up, she patted my shoulder approvingly. I was on top of the world. What a break-through!

During my first year as a volunteer, I was eager to help, and scared to try. Thankfully, my skills increased over time, so I was given more projects to do independently. Eventually, I increased time spent at BIAM from one to two days. As I felt my self-confidence return, I experienced a kind of euphoria. It became easier to feel proud of my accomplishments. When I was a cost accountant in the apparel industry, I usually felt insignificant - I was in it mostly for the paycheck. As a volunteer for a small, non-profit organization, I could more easily view the larger picture, while working on my corner of it. It was then that I began to feel essential.

My phone skills increased dramatically. I could still get flustered when too many calls happened at one time, but I was proud of each one handled. There was real exhilaration for me when I heard a voice on the phone change from despair to cheerfulness, just because I gave him or her a few minutes of my time. When I informed the caller that I am also a survivor of brain injury, I could sometimes hear their incredulous wonder, which also lifted my spirits. I have never before been symbolic of hope and possibilities. And I thank God for leading me to the brain injury community where I am needed.

Prior to joining the Brain Injury Association of Maryland, I searched my local library for information about brain injury. Some of the books were too technical, therefore too challenging for someone without sound reading comprehension. At BIAM, I fully indulged in self-education. The choices seemed endless. I discovered fascinating and informative material as I explored the filing cabinets and shelves. My changed reading skills were being thoroughly satisfied with the choices available. Today I am much better informed about this mysterious injury within my skull, and to have a better understanding of my brain injury has removed some of the sting.

Another favorite activity was discovering written material to copy and make available to the association's visitors. As someone on the "inside", I think that I had a good sense of what would appeal to others like me. When spending time at the copy machine, it was not always easy to be aware that I was contributing to the mission of BIAM. Except that, when I saw the copies in the hands of survivors, their families, providers, or the public, I knew that I contributed an essential piece of the puzzle. In addition, when I saw an interested passer-by drawn to a display that I had just replenished, I was convinced that my time has been well spent.

Suddenly, a simple administrative task was elevated to a high level of importance.

When I noticed visitors gathered around our hall display, I joined them. As they perused the choices and picked out some to keep, I mentally noted what seemed popular. Sometimes they exclaimed aloud about the good material available, and I was proud to have provided it. These were also opportunities to present myself to the loved ones of patients on the brain injury unit of Kernan Hospital. Their obvious grief and worried expressions provoked my empathy. I felt a very strong desire to ease their pain and to offer hope. These bewildered family members frequently said the same thing. "_____ has a brain injury, but I don't know what that means."

It is very disturbing that such a potentially devastating injury is still shrouded in mystery. The Brain Injury Association of Maryland is seeking to educate the public about this extremely prevalent occurrence. Did you know that every year over 6 thousand Marylanders join the TBI club (CDC 2006)? BIAM receives no government funds. They depend entirely upon grants, sponsorship, and membership to continue their good work.

Recently, I bumped into a family arriving at the brain injury unit to visit their loved one. I had met the man previously. He had told me about his severely injured daughter, and that she was not responding very well. He seemed entirely without hope, then. When I saw him again, he introduced me to other family members as an example of hope. We approached the door to the gym on the unit, opened it, and stood gaping at the incredible scene. The young woman in question was on her feet and taking tentative steps with the help of a caring physical therapist. She was wearing an awkward assortment of fixtures to stabilize parts of her body, but still trying. We all were overcome with emotion, but I retreated as they joined their loved one. I recalled my own experiences as a patient in that gym.

I was a volunteer. It was my answer to the question, what do you do? The four words described a career paradoxically draining and fulfilling, charitable and self-seeking. For four years, I had happily volunteered with the Brain Injury Association of Maryland. This worthy organization exists to improve the lives of my people and me. So why are we still not state or federally funded? What better opportunity for state and federal government to prove that they are truly of *all* the people, by *all* the people, and for *all* the people?

On a typical day, I handled a dozen or more telephone calls, posted and retrieved the mail, made photocopies, replenished displays, researched on the internet and offered support to families visiting us from the brain injury unit at Kernan Hospital. BIAM is a significant resource for the hospital. I was never bored, but sometimes I felt overwhelmed. After a good night's sleep, I could start eagerly, with plenty of energy, but fatigue overtook me suddenly, at the end of my day. The evidence was diminished cognitive functions like: slower thinking, being less organized, being more forgetful, becoming less articulate, and crankier behavior.

One of the most uplifting activities was the privilege to talk with someone like me or their loved one. In all the years as an accountant, I do not remember a moment of absolute certainty that my existence made a difference. Now, I am often treated to this thrilling revelation. To hear the voice of a caller change from despondent to optimistic was tonic for my occasional depression. Who would have thought that my value to humanity would *increase* because of brain injury?

Internet research can be tedious. However, I have found that it is a task worth doing, because some very important reasons occur to me. One is that it is a primary source of education for me about the many aspects of brain injury. Another is brain exercise. Working memory, sequencing, problem solving, and reading comprehension are just some of the exercises. In addition, I get a share in educating the public about brain injury.

Special projects are a good source of practical vocational experience for me. With the approach of our tenth annual Eat A Peach Challenge Bike Ride, came a daunting mountain of work. I was not responsible for the bulk of it, however. BIAM's brilliant and enduring assistant director, Suzanne Kantt, was. Thanks to her, this very important prevention focused outreach fundraiser is more successful every year.

The portion of the tasks that were mine are as follows: gather and coordinate a crew of volunteer help (about 60 individuals), alert the media, and find donations of food, paper products and supplies for a picnic lunch. The volunteers were from the brain injury community, professionals, and providers who work with family members, friends, and neighbors. I have the utmost respect for all of them. They continue to be an essential element to the success of the bike ride. If you are wondering about the name, Eat A Peach, we share quarters with the August Peach Festival at the Agricultural Center in Westminster, Maryland.

As I handled the emails, phone calls, and letter writing, I always encountered one of the most frustrating and misunderstood aspects of brain injury - fatigue. I have clear memory of engaging in activities like the ones described above every day pre-injury, tirelessly, and without second thoughts. Now the effects of over-extending myself have become an expectation. Comprehension of the huge amount of energy required just to think is mine.

Do not wait to acquire a brain injury for comprehension to become yours. Believe what you cannot see. My intense anger is raised when I hear of the extremely unjust use of the word, malingerer, to describe me or one of my fellow walking wounded. I have even been accused by a close relative of just seeking pity! Can you believe it?

The Brain Injury Association of Maryland organizes and presents an annual two-day educational conference. It was at one of these conferences that I met Trisha Meili; author of I Am the Central Park Jogger. She was our keynote speaker. Prior to the conference I had read her book and was truly excited to meet her. We sat together at a book-signing event the day before the conference and became friends. I will never forget the gentleness and intelligence of this courageous woman. She inspired me to never give up hope, and I treasure the few letters that we have shared. Another author who was keynote speaker for BIAM at the conference was Jackie Pflug. She wrote, <u>Miles to go Before I Sleep</u>. Her story is about surviving a terrorist attack on a hijacked plane, during which she was shot in the head. Her riveting story lifted my spirits, too, just when I needed to know that it is possible to have a happy and productive life after acquiring a brain injury. Diane Triplett has honored me with the request to be the keynote speaker at the April 2010 conference. I have accepted. I hope that I can do as well as the speakers that I have heard.

A few years ago, my duties included planning and running a breakout session. It was an informal gathering of survivors to discuss two topics of my choice. It was a parlor session, which I named, <u>Second Wind</u>, after the Billy Joel song, and I was honored with the responsibility. Who would have thought, that three years after joining BIAM, the opportunity would be mine? When they first knew me, I was very withdrawn and anxious. Dr. Hopkins still teases me about being scared to answer the phone. So you see, recovery can and does happen and it continues over time.

I started the one-hour session with a brief reading of excerpts from a short memoir I had written during the previous year. That memoir is contained entirely within this book. We discussed disinhibition versus self-control and on-the-job fatigue. I was gratified by the willing discussion that was sometimes intense. The hour flew by, and in the end, I enjoyed the warm praise of Mark Huslage, about the success of the session. He is a social worker who runs the Return! Program at Sinai Hospital in Baltimore; and he was present, if needed. Mark's unwavering good nature has always been a pleasure.

The rest of the conference was a series of presentations and discussions of all of the following and more: the benefits of physical exercise, education, medications, sleep disorders, depression, personality changes, behavior management, therapies for independence, mild TBI, stroke rehabilitation, Social Security, and cognitive rehabilitation and remediation. We also offered a two-day review session and exam by the American Academy for the Certification of Brain Injury Specialists. There were breakout sessions by other survivors or family members to present and discuss their personal experiences with brain injury. We are suitably proud of our months of hard work to present such a comprehensive conference. Explain to me again, why we are not state or federally funded?

This experience reminded me of my own diminished stamina. Furthermore, I discovered, again, that I can have a significant effect on others both symbolically and practically - a very important lesson for me. The huge expenditure of energy was worth it. My breakout session was a revelation that turned out to be the catalyst urging me to arrange for something similar, but permanent. I needed to form a support group in my part of the state where one did not exist.

Support Group

During my time at BIAM, I had been encouraged to start a support group. Even Dr. Hopkins had mentioned it once or twice. My initial reaction was absolutely not, because my self-confidence was low and my trepidation high. After three more years of recovery, I was finally ready. First, I read and reread <u>Helping Ourselves, A Guide for Brain Injury Support Groups</u>, a Brain Injury Association, Inc. publication that has been very helpful. My still unreliable reading comprehension requires occasional study of this book for cognitive refreshment. It is not that I am a poorer student post-injury, but that new learning is harder work for me. However, I have not lost my high degree of curiosity. I was looking forward to being both the leader and the facilitator, but anxious about handling the meetings alone. My husband came to my rescue again. He graciously offered to be my partner in the venture, and with over thirty years experience as a nurse, he was superbly qualified. I feel stronger and more confident in his company.

My associates at the Brain Injury Association of Maryland were very helpful and excited about the support group. Suzanne Kantt researched our database. Then, volunteers mailed out flyers to the extensive list of individuals in and around my area. I sent public service announcements to the local papers and set up an information display at my parish church where the meetings are held. I also sent a quantity of announcements to my contact at the public library headquarters. She offered to distribute them to all of the branches in my county. I began to compile a list of emails and phone messages from interested parties.

As I set up the room for our first meeting, Mike was making coffee in the very handy nearby kitchen. Curiously, the room seemed to have changed greatly and hardly at all since I last used it. I was at St. Joseph's Catholic Community in Eldersburg, Carroll County, Maryland. They graciously lent us a room for the monthly meetings. More than twenty five years earlier, I had been a CCD (Sunday school) teacher. I prepared lesson plans to share with eleven-year-olds on Sundays. The rows of desks and chairs and the old-fashioned chalkboard were gone. Instead, four large tables formed a solid fixture in the middle of the room, surrounded by seating for fifteen adults. There was a smaller, white, dry-erase board on a sidewall and a freestanding easel on the opposite side. The comforting sight of youthful classroom art decorating the back wall took me back through the years.

I remembered a favorite activity and display. My sixth graders authored personal messages to Jesus and rolled them small enough to fit into slits on a cardboard scene attached to the back wall. The scene was two shores on opposite sides of a painted body of water with slits at the ends of bobbing bottles. On one shore was a crowd of youngsters, each claimed with a name of one of my students. On the opposite shore was a smiling Jesus, stooping to retrieve the messages in bottles. Jim Croce's <u>Time in a Bottle</u> played while we worked on this project.

I swallowed the lump in my throat as my support group members wandered in, one with a quad-cane, one in a wheelchair, still others with careful, deliberate gate. How can life change so drastically and not at all in 25 years? I wanted so badly to provide comfort and hope to my people. As I looked into their troubled and expectant faces, I felt my usual rush of empathy. They were just like me. We settled down for our first meeting. The

collection of spirals on the table was claimed one by one. My own love of journalizing and writing prompted me to suggest that they each use a spiral to record their thoughts and feelings. I collected and saved the spirals to bring to every meeting. Over time, each one of us can read and discover how we have changed. The significant life-change over which none of us had control can be contrasted with our own personal achievements. We can treat ourselves to pats on the back, because we are doing just fine. We spent two hours together, during which time, we shared, cried, and laughed. All the administrative preparation led to an inspiring evening. As I bade each individual goodnight, I hoped that they also were proud of where they are because of where they had been.

Brain Injury + Responsibility = Growth

Why is dog ownership recommended for persons with disability? It is recommended for the same reason that exercise is recommended for everyone with and without disability - young, middle-aged, and old.

Exercise is for improved health. A healthy body can better withstand life's traumas and illnesses. An essential part of your physical body is hidden within your skull. Your brain is another one of your body's organs - like your liver, heart, or kidneys. It can be injured, too. Oxygen is essential for life. Living organisms thrive when oxygenated. We are living organisms - every inch of us. Exercise not only increases and strengthens muscle tissue and bone density, it also oxygenates your body. To keep a plentiful and steady flow of oxygen going to your brain keeps it alive, helps it to recover from injury, and helps it to fight disease. I am at my cognitive sharpest when my exercise routine is vigorous and regular. A pleasing aesthetic side effect is also welcome - a healthy, toned body.

When recovering from brain injury, certain psychological issues may need to be addressed. I have discussed professional counseling, which I strongly recommend. Did you know that it is possible to exercise your psyche, too? What is the single most important factor for anyone's psychological maturation and growth? My personal answer is *responsibility*. I apologize if I am not discussing your answer. To be responsible for the welfare of another living thing can hasten the maturation process. What does that have to do with brain injury? Maturity is not something we are born with. We learn it over time and store it in our brains. When injury to that organ occurs, much of what we have learned can be lost. It is the reason why therapists must teach their patients basic functionality - walking, talking, and feeding oneself, how to do personal care, reading, writing, and math. That part of my recovery, although factual, is lost in amnesia.

My husband saw an opportunity to satisfy two needs with one acquisition. He got the dog that he had always wanted, and provided an opportunity for growth for me. I accepted added responsibility, and the chance to return Mike's love through caring for his dog. We named the dog Cooper, after the surgeon who saved my life. Cooper was a handsome, intelligent animal who responded well to training. He was my walking companion, and helped me to come out of my shell. There is nothing like a good dog to encourage socializing in one's neighborhood.

I was not always comfortable with the extra work, though. I

experienced resentment and anger when I had concluded that I was being taken advantage of. I hate housework; I would like to do it once, and have it stay clean for a long time. At other times, especially after dark, the presence of another warm body makes me feel less lonely. In addition, the relationship with a dog is less complicated than with another person. The animal is always loyal, loving, forgiving, and accepting. Cooper and I enjoyed long walks in the cornfield across from our house, and in the wooded area beyond. We also enjoyed exploring the watershed area with Mike, about one mile from home. Ultimately, I loved having Cooper around.

On January 1, 2005, I was working on a poem that I had started before Christmas. Cooper slept peacefully at my feet. Later that night, I took the dog for a walk in my neighborhood. I made the unfortunate decision not to leash him. On the way back from the walk, he spotted and chased an unknown animal into the road and was killed instantly. I am still horrified by the memory, and bear a huge amount of guilt. I dedicate "One Mile from Home" to our dear Cooper.

One Mile from Home
A menacing sky,
a sink full of dishes,
Cooper needs walking,
so does his lady.

So damn the snow
and the dishes.
Come on dog

it's our turn.

We pass below trees that tap
each other's shoulders,
and an acrobatic chipmunk
puts on a show.

From tree to tree
chatty sparrows flit,
shrubs shake off
quarreling cardinals.

Grazing deer one mile distant,
framed by trees, seem near.
Cooper gazes expectantly,
but the trail beckons.

Onward to a leaden lake
hardening silently
while snowflakes stick themselves
to skin and fur.

Home is sanctuary
and obligations wait
something dark stares
from a vultured tree
at our backs.

December 2004

Counseling

The sixth anniversary of my first meeting with Dr. William Hopkins has happened. It feels as if I have known "Bill" all of my life - since childhood. Although we have met and talked almost 300 times, we have not run out of topics to discuss. Our conversations are usually one-sided, though. I do most of the talking, and Dr. Hopkins does most of the listening.

I believe that I made a very good decision to follow the advice of two neuropsychologists -- Dr. Vince Culotta and Dr. Mark Sementilli. Talk therapy has been good for me. I am also convinced that the longevity of the relationship is mostly due to the congeniality of Dr. William Hopkins. But our relationship is not always a happy one. We have had very serious disagreements that resulted in my taking a sabbatical. However, I always return for more good therapy.

The benefits of counseling for me are as follows: a. self-discovery, b. support, c. problem solving, d. growth, and e. healing. It is impossible for me to predict how much longer I will seek counseling with Dr. Hopkins. It seems like we still have a lot of work to do. This book was actually suggested by Bill, and he has been very supportive while I have written it. The following is his contribution, in the form of answers to my questions.

> How long have you known Eileen? *I first met Eileen on February 7, 2001.*

> What is your earliest memory of her? *The admonition "Don't call me Grace!" comes readily*

to mind. I recall Eileen being very articulate, even in her initial session just four months following her traumatic brain injury. Her occasional struggle to find the precise words she wanted to use did not obscure her obvious intelligence and emerging insight into the challenges she faced. Still there were also signs of disinhibition that occasionally allowed strong emotion to interfere with her reasoning.

What was your assessment of her then? *She was embarking on the daunting path of rediscovering herself. To me, her "scenarios" represented both a determined effort to reconstruct a fuller memory of her early days of recovery and to explore the new person she was becoming. Lingering grief and anger provided a sobering context for this journey. The stark realities of her cognitive impairments, her physical scars, the loss of her career, and the changes in her impulse control and personality triggered periods of despondency and intense anger and resentment. These were understandable stages in the psychological process of her recovery.*

Did it occur to you that the relationship might be a long one? *I knew that the relationship might be a sustained one because she was expecting much of herself and her recovery.*

Has Eileen progressed since you've known her? How? *On an emotional level, Eileen has progressed substantially. Her disinhibition has remitted and she has moved through her grief and anger enough to reclaim control of her life. Cognitively, her working memory has also improved, although it remains significantly below her capacity prior to her traumatic brain injury. Short term memory flaws are still evident as well, though less frequent. Emerging out of these changes is her discovery of a new sense of purpose. The determination and commitment she displayed throughout her work in therapy have contributed much to her success as a volunteer at the Brain Injury Association of Maryland and as a leader for a support group.*

What are the contributing factors to her progress? *The support of her husband has proved vital along her course in recovery. He has encouraged her to pursue therapy at difficult and painful junctures and has provided a nurturing presence when her grief and anger overwhelmed her. Also, the determination she developed in childhood has enabled her to persist despite daily reminders of how her life has changed permanently in virtually every respect. Curiously, some of the personality changes associated with her brain injury have lent themselves to her substantial recovery as well. A more open communication style has helped her to overcome her sense of distance enough to forge bonds with others that have broadened her support network. A heightened sense of compassion has helped motivate her to design a new purpose for her life through her work with other brain injury survivors. And fortunately for Eileen, she has retained a high level of intelligence that empowers her to pursue her ongoing plans through recovery, including her current writing project.*

What are some highlights of your time together? Lowlights? *The most prominent highlight in my mind was her decision to volunteer at BIAM. This represented a significant move beyond the grief that had consumed her and a return to the world that could, in turn, provide the opportunity for her to rediscover a sense of purpose and restore her self esteem. The lowlights generally involved an occasional tendency for her to interpret rifts in the therapeutic rapport as confirmation of her fear that others would see and treat her as a victim.*

Have you treated other persons with brain injury? *While not an area of specialization, I have treated a number of people with brain injuries through my work in nursing homes and outpatient settings.*

What are the aspects of brain injury survivors that makes it easier or more difficult to treat them? *In my experience, the strategy varies by the relative skills of each survivor. Some have retained capacity for more ambitious therapy involving grief and the difficult readjustment to their lives while others*

*function at a more concrete cognitive level or lack
adequate short term memory and respond better to
behavioral interventions.*

Have there been any breakthroughs with Eileen?
Like what? *In my opinion, there have been several
breakthroughs that were crucial to her recovery. First,
she was able to relinquish much of her anger towards
the driver primarily responsible for her injuries
through forgiveness. Next, she was able to overcome
her fixation on physical scars thanks in part to the
efforts of Dr. Singh. She then had to abandon her
stubborn insistence that she would not return to work
at a position that was less demanding than her career
in accounting. That involved ultimate acceptance of
her residual cognitive deficits, a difficult prospect for
a determined woman who had taken pride in her
professional accomplishments.*

What are her strengths? Weaknesses? *Her strengths
with regard to her recovery include: her open and
articulate style of communication; her largely intact
verbal reasoning; her determination and persistence;
her desire to forge relationships despite the sense
of distance from others that has plagued her since
her brain injury; and her sense of humor. Her
weaknesses include: some residual tendency to obsess
about disturbing incidents; strong emotions that can
compromise her ability to reason; a diminished ability
to manage multiple tasks simultaneously; faults in*

short term memory.

What have you learned from Eileen? *I have learned how resilient the therapeutic bond can be with a brain injured client even when intense, focused anger interrupts the process. I have also felt privileged to witness the transformation she has wrought through the course of grieving her losses and rebuilding her sense of purpose through reaching out to others.*

What is your opinion of the book she is writing? *I applaud her decision to write a book. In my opinion, this project is a logical extension of both her desire to help others by sharing her experience and of her process of self discovery that she embarked upon through her "scenarios."*

If you could, what would you provide for all brain injury survivors? *If I could (and I am not claiming that I can), I would provide them with the tools needed to restore primary relationships and to recover a sense of engagement and purpose in life.* When is it time to end this relationship? *In my mind, the end to a relationship is the result of an ongoing dialog, a mutual process. I expect that the therapeutic relationship will conclude when Eileen and I agree that she has gained optimally from the experience Her attempt to run a BI support group seems a natural extension of her work at BIAM. Through her efforts in the BI community with survivors and their families, she has found a renewed sense of worth and purpose that had eluded her in the earlier phases of her recovery when grief and resentment about her lost career had preoccupied and hampered her.*

Exiled...

"That's the time you must keep on trying. Smile; what's the use of crying? You'll find that life is still worthwhile, if you'll just smile."
-Charlie Chaplin

Since I acquired a brain injury, I have been plagued by a feeling of separation from humanity and from myself. Clinicians call this condition, *Loss of Self*. This frightfully lonely feeling has taken many forms, but I will try to illustrate the sensation in this chapter.

It seems like everyone is moving forward, except me. I am constantly left behind, exhausted by the effort of trying to catch up. I do not equate the phenomenon with any particular malice, but I am certain that it is related to my reduced cognitive abilities. Being held back by some unseen shackle prevents me from keeping up.

Imagine, for a moment, a business meeting on any subject. Colleagues are gathered to discuss researched information on topics from previous meetings and to introduce new topics. This normal and harmless activity requires interpersonal skills, flexible thinking, good working memory, prioritizing, note taking, and sound comprehension. If you have deficits in any of these areas, the meeting can move along at light speed, but without you. The loneliness, anger, and resentment that you may feel, can lead you to believe that your colleagues are being thoughtless, when they are not.

Have you ever been in a zoo, viewing the ape-like creatures? Have you lingered at the chimpanzee exhibit? Think about picking out the individuals as they go about their business - some are eating - some are napping - some are socializing - some are cavorting and showing off their acrobatic skills. You may notice that although they have similarities, they are not duplicates of each other. You may begin to realize that they each have a unique look, and that they have different behaviors and attitudes. Perhaps their different personalities are apparent, even though their brains are much smaller than ours. They are covered with hair, except for their faces, hands, and feet. Did you know that, just like with humans, these are concentrated centers for the senses? A young chimp might take an interest in you, and gaze at you with innocence and surprisingly intelligent curiosity. The youngster might reach out his long arm toward you, and maybe you respond naturally, extending your hand toward him. With a bemused expression upon your face, you expect to shake hands with him, but instead you encounter a glass partition. You cannot touch him. Are you disappointed?

Do you remember where you were on September 11, 2001? How did you feel? Perhaps you experienced shock, horror, grief, anger, and a little post-traumatic stress. Were you completely absorbed by the unbelievable scenes; glued to the television? Were you so moved by all the horrible death and destruction that you had to hold back tears? As you watched all the news coverage, and the obvious emotions of the seasoned veteran reporters and anchors, what was your reaction? Were your interpersonal relationships affected? Maybe the scope of the tragedy caused you to draw closer to your loved ones. I suspect that you also felt very strongly a part of the great team of the United States - more patriotic. What if you realized that your feelings and reactions were different from everyone else's? Suppose you couldn't feel anything, and were afraid to let anyone see? What would you conclude about yourself? How about - you have nothing in common with the rest of humanity?

Loss of Self

Let us talk about familiarity. Do you have a favorite chair? Is it always your choice for seating, when in that room? Regardless of the chair style, wooden or stuffed, are you relieved to lower yourself into it? If you are in it now, notice how much pleasure you feel. Maybe the act of gazing around at the familiar setting generates a warm feeling of home. When you are away from home, do you sometimes long for what is familiar?

Now let us expand our consideration to the place we call home. When in it, we revel in a level of comfort not found anywhere else. Compare the two distinct feelings experienced when leaving your home and when returning to it. Perhaps you undergo regret followed by relief. Have you ever wondered why you feel so comfortable in your own home? Maybe it is because you can be yourself. Certain behaviors and habits are acceptable in your familiar environment. Maybe, that is why we feel compelled to go through a preparation ritual to leave home. Many survivors of brain injury struggle with a phenomenon called "loss of self." When you become aware that your formerly familiar personal setting has undergone significant change unexpectedly, a myriad of questions may rise to the surface: Why? What? When?

Where? How? If the personal setting is you - your brain, then the bewildered expletive might be, "Huh?" Extreme comfort with my own brain and body was something I took for granted, until it was lost. Now I feel like there is a bus depot inside of me.

Let us ponder this too. To have an out-of-body experience is desirable. This extremely pleasurable sensation can more easily happen when your body and mind are completely relaxed. I have experienced this wonder a few times in my life, and I have found it to be quite enjoyable. Some practiced individuals know how to cause it to happen at their will. I am not one of them. For me, it was completely unexpected, when I was on the verge of sleep, and over quickly. It felt like I was lifted up and out of my own body, which stayed behind. The separation was painless, but I felt like I was divided into two beings - one weightless - one weighted. The curious floating feeling that followed was something to look forward to. When I rejoined my body, it was like the gentle landing of a falling leaf. Suppose you awake to find yourself outside of your body, but you cannot get back in? Where would you go? Do you think that you would be scared and bewildered?

Now let's consider the possibility of having all three of these sensations at the same time, A) A barrier exists between you and everyone else, B) You frequently feel completely different from everyone - like another species, and C) You are disconnected from yourself. The extreme understatement that this is a disturbing situation is full of sick humor. Having these perceptions, together or separately, can generate loneliness, depression, desperation, and high anxiety. If you feel all of the above at the same time, do you think that your behavior might reflect the emotional trauma? I have just provided an answer to another question frequently asked of me. Why do you need psycho-therapy for your brain injury?

To reminisce - pleasurable, is it not? Who doesn't like to relax with old friends over coffee and talk about the past? Mr. Webster describes it, most charmingly as, recalling bygone experiences. Put yourself in a scene on a velvety summer night on a patio, deck, or porch. Maybe candles flicker in jars, and there are competing choruses of crickets, locusts, and tree frogs. The night-bloomers fragrantly glow in the dark, and fireflies flash each other, adding to the magic. Scents from the delicious meal you just shared still linger.

Everyone lounges comfortably, replete and content. Conversation begins languidly about the food, the drink, and the day that just ended. You have known each other many years and have witnessed mutual youth become maturity. Life's experiences show on your faces and bodies, except for one person's significant life-change that is present and invisible. Familiarity enables the group to have immediate recall, with cues consisting of just one or two words. Then, lively, fast-paced hilarity proceeds. Perhaps, original events have been obscured under layers of embellishment over the years, making them even funnier. But your laughter may be more forced than everyone else's.

Occasionally, someone may look at you curiously. The smile on your face can begin to feel like a mask and your forehead suddenly has a sensation like you just walked into a door. The strange twitchiness in your legs that keeps you awake at night begins and your face burns where the scar is, like an electrical shock. The annoying sensation of scampering critters inside your skull makes you put your fingers through your hair to rub your scalp vigorously. One of your guests asks kindly, "Are you okay?" With as much grace as you can muster, you answer, "I'm fine, thank you." What a lie you just told! Conversation continues around you, but mostly without you. Your contributions are in the form of a high-pitched hysterical-sounding giggle. Where did that come from? You would like to express your thoughts, but they come very slowly when everyone else has moved to another topic. When you do insert your voice, it sounds slow, measured, and serious. Why can't you be funny?

Your friends start many stories like this, "Remember that day in Social Studies? Remember that guy in the sweater? Remember that day on the parking lot? Remember when Williamson got mad at us?" *If* you remember what *they* do, your recall is much slower and certain details never surface at all. Silently, you scream, "Slow down!"Occasionally, a question is shot your way, but while you are still searching for the answer, the group moves on. Maybe the blank expression on your face elicits curious looks from the others. Discouraged, you subside silently to observe and listen from the outside. Your detachment grows as you try to understand why you are no longer interested in the conversation. Perhaps your mind begins to wander as you cease paying attention to the others. Questions may come to your mind such as, "When did they change so much? What is their hurry? Why isn't their company interesting anymore?"

Under these circumstances, it would be so easy to conclude

that they do not care about you because your isolation is complete. Should you have answered your friend's question, "Are you okay?" more honestly? You would have brought up the same old tired subject of the effects of brain injury, and has that not become boring? Also, during past attempts to make your situation understood, you seem to have failed. Moreover, why should your friends have to behave differently? They did not do anything wrong.

When the evening breaks up, the group departs, still laughing. They almost seem energized by the encounter, but your own fatigue is defeating. You also cannot understand why you are suddenly on the verge of tears. Your companions do not notice, however, because a stupid smile is still pasted on your face.

The way to recovery is not a clear track upon which one makes steady, forward progress. All of humanity is on this life course together. We begin at the same point, and then proceed to the inevitable finish line. For those on the primary track, the way is clear. So, the footrace is unobstructed. I was transferred to track two as of October 3, 2000.

Did you ever race hurdles, maybe in your youth? I was lousy at it. How about you? But the choice is no longer mine and now I struggle to continue my forward progress. It seems like I need twice the energy to go half the distance. Am I losing ground? The struggle to keep up with my former teammates can leave me crumpled in despair at the base of another hurdle. I am sometimes unable to get up and try again, due to crushing fatigue. The hurdles are not consistent in size or distance from each other. What they have in common, though, is that they are all barriers. They keep me apart from my former teammates.

To successfully clear a hurdle is certainly something to celebrate, but you will see it again. Brain injury is a chronic condition. Once you have it, you take it with you wherever you go for the rest of your life. There is no cure. Check out this list of typical effects of brain injury. If you had to cope with some or all of the following items every day, your emotional well being would be in jeopardy.

❑   Attention Deficit. *You cannot focus on one thing for a specific amount of time.*

❑   Distractibility. *You cannot stay focused when there is other noise or activity present.*

❑   Initiation/Completion Deficit. *You cannot get started on or finish any task or project.*

❑   Planning and Sequencing Deficit. *You cannot create a logical, organized plan of action for even a simple task.*

❑   Poor Judgment and Perception. *You cannot interpret actions or intentions of others and you may have an unrealistic self-appraisal.*

❑   Memory Deficit. *You have trouble learning new information, and may have trouble retrieving old information.*

❑   Slower processing speed. *You have difficulty*

keeping up with "normal" conversation; a movie plot; a television show; a news story; driving in heavy traffic; or answering questions

❑ Communication Deficit. *You may not comprehend the conversation of others, or "find" the right words for self-expression.*

❑ Disinhibition. *No social censor; impulsive; lack of self-control.*

❑ Emotionally Labile. *Severe mood swings. Maybe you get too angry. Maybe you cry too much.*

❑ Fatigue. *Sudden, defeating, subduing, conquering.*

❑ Depression *Annoying, chronic, and dangerous.*

You may have concluded that since I share these very common effects with others like me, there is companionship in brain injury. Truthfully, when we are in each other's company, we can feel more socially accepted. It is not difficult for me to be kind, understanding, and patient with others like me. When we part, however, I am acutely and immediately aware of being isolated in my own bubble of dysfunction. Moreover, the worst feeling of clinical depression is profound loneliness. It is possible to have close relationships, to touch, or to be part of a crowd without making a connection. It is as if an electric shortage has occurred and the connection is severed.

Depression

Depression is the one hurdle that truly frightens me. Is there a limit to how many times one can overcome this menace? I have lost count of the number of times that I have been tripped by the meanest hurdle of all. Many BI survivors turn to drugs and alcohol for solace. They have my complete understanding and my compassion. If I knew how to end my pain, I would share the knowledge with others in the brain injury community. I am thinking, especially, of a former classmate of mine and Mike's. He sustained a mild traumatic brain injury from an accident with a chain saw while helping a neighbor. Soon after, he was tormented by seizures and memory issues. Different treatments were prescribed but nothing helped and then he was terminated from his job. Suicide was how our friend ended his anguish and Mike and I were severely shaken. The seriousness of depression should never be underestimated.

To be so far from life is truly scary. The further away I get, the harder it is to come back. Depression is a barrier between me and everyone else, including family. Tragically, when Mike and I get into arguments, we point the finger at each other too much, when brain injury is really to blame. Mike tells me that I am too sensitive, that I focus too long on one subject, and that I am too emotional. He is correct. These effects of brain injury still burden me after years of therapy, and I don't know if I will ever have the maturity and self control that I need. Mike is also affected by brain injury because of the changes in his spouse. If he can find a way to accept these changes instead of allowing himself to become so annoyed with me, that would help me to stay calm. From my side of the glass between us, there is sometimes agonizing sadness, hopelessness, pessimism, and emotional trauma. From his side of the glass between us, he probably notices fewer smiles, more tears, less laughter, less patience, withdrawal, and resentment. Who would not be turned off, maybe angered by such a display? I understand his anger. Frequent bouts of depression can drive families apart.

Interpersonal relationships

Maintaining old or establishing new interpersonal relationships is by far the most troublesome aspect of my recovery. The intrusiveness of BI is burdensome, persistent, and annoying. My unreliable memory causes more trouble between me and my husband than you can imagine. If I am making a sandwich for Mike, he must repeat his preferences more than once to me. But I may still forget and have to ask him again. If he reminds me about a chore that I still need to do but I don't accomplish the task immediately, the slightest distraction can erase it from my mind entirely. Another culprit is comprehension deficit. Mike and I can be having a conversation about anything such as, a television show or a movie. As he speaks, Mike can leave me far behind, because he is a much quicker thinker than I am. Too often, I need him to repeat what he has said in order to form and express my own opinion. Then, the double dilemma of not understanding either Mike or the broadcast can cause conflict between us. It is as if we no longer speak the same language. One of the worst characteristics of BI for me is the volatile mixture of my hypersensitivity and over emotionalism. The slightest misunderstanding between us can lead to thoughtless remarks, which I take very personally. Then I feel slighted and hurt, which can lead to an emotional outburst and tears. Living with me can be like being a porcupine trying to safely cross a field of balloons. I, on the other hand, feel like a kite in a thunderstorm. My brain injury is not obvious because I have a normal presentation. Therefore, it is very hard for Mike to form new habits that are suitable for a relationship with the new me. What is difficult for me is to relax and to believe in Mike's continued devotion to me, even though I have changed. Nevertheless, we must both try; love is worth fighting for. Here are my suggestions:

For the family

- Find professional counseling for you and your loved one; preferably, someone experienced with brain injury.

- Stay calm. Try not to lose your temper. Raised voices and mean words will make your loved one withdraw more.

- Try to keep your own complaints to a minimum. Avoid expressing disappointments in your loved one. A person with BI can have very low self-esteem.

- Accentuate the positive. Minimize the negative. Let your loved one see your pleasure in him/her.

For the person with brain injury

- Don't sweat the small stuff. Keep reminding yourself what is really important in your life. Do not spend time and energy on what is not.

- Remember your love. You have a lot to give. Don't be stingy with your family.

- Keep your faith. You are here because you have work to do, and the world is better because you are in it.

- Your recovery is within reach. Go get it.

Brain Injury + Amnesia = Loss of Self

An unbroken line of memory is a normal part of being human. A fun and interesting exercise is to trace your life in the form of a time line.

Birth, Childhood, Montreal	High School, South Carroll	Marriage 1971	Career, Accountant	Carroll Community College

You now have a visual representation of your life as a solid, structured, logical progression. No matter how many factors you insert, the connections on your time line are not severed. Your life is a continuous ribbon, the length of which is unknown. Point to any part of your time line, except birth, and you become connected to it by memory. You have created an answer to the question, "Who am I?" Your answer is accessible and complete due to memory. As you gaze at this personal graph with affectionate interest, you may become aware of a feeling of security because you know who you are. The evidence is before you.

Try an experiment. Cut a year/event section off of your time line and discard it like it never happened.

Birth, Childhood, Montreal	High School, South Carroll	Marriage 1971		Carroll Community College

Consider the severed ends of what is left. Does it take considerable repair to reconnect the two ends? Perhaps you also notice that the progression of your life is no longer smooth and even. The step-by-step logical pattern seems to be missing something. Try using a blank section as a connector piece. Does a blank make more or less sense in your time line? What is the memory that connects you to the blank? Your answer to the question, "Who am I?" is now represented by the reconstructed time line. Perhaps the answer is now unclear, and you feel compelled to offer an explanation for the gap and reconstruction.

When amnesia becomes part of your life, you continue, but not as before. Holding together the severed ends of ones life can be labor intensive and exhausting. It is easy to feel disconnected from your life without the glue of memory. The metamorphosis of your life, part A, to your life, part B, is concealed within a cocoon of amnesia. You know, factually, that certain events occurred, but the sequence is invisible. It is possible to have some unknown acquaintances. Individuals who serviced you with critical and intimate care may forever be strangers. The size of the blank section on your time line may not accurately represent the enormity of the processes that formed the current you. It can also be hard to accept that during the time of amnesia, you may have participated in important activities. What did you do? Whom did you talk to? You may even wonder about your behavior. Was it appropriate?

Before driving you all the way to insanity, please consider a couple of facts. A) You cannot retrieve what does not exist. The recording device in your brain was switched off at the time of amnesia. B) It is a fact of life for all humans that we begin our lives with some amnesia. We cannot remember birth, infancy, and very early childhood. Many of us have reached our fourth or fifth birthdays before our brain's recording device is fully functional.

As a survivor of brain injury, which includes amnesia, I understand that the facts can be hard to accept. I am still working on finding a level of comfort with what I cannot change. With the help of my experienced counselor and my devoted husband and family, I am making excellent progress. Remember, that in nature, a thing of beauty can eventually emerge from a cocoon and take flight.

Amnesia is not only a solid and definitive portion of time without memory. It can also be a small, unexpected blank spot within a filled space. The solid ribbon that represents the time line of one's life can be severed by coma, but it can also resemble a damaged motion picture.

Cookware Party

I knew her face, her name, and her voice. She was very familiar, but how did I know her? As I chose a muffin for my plate from the table full of goodies, I became aware of her by my side. She said, "How are you, Eileen?" Did I detect irony in her voice, or am I nuts? "Very well, Sylvia, how are you?" I chirped in my best fake-normal voice with matching smile. My interest in the rest of the goodies waned, and I found a seat apart from the group. A dryness in my throat developed when I glanced at the familiar stranger. My thoughtful daughter kindly brought me a drink.

I felt separate from the group of women gathered for a cookware demonstration. While they joked and exclaimed over which products to buy, I retreated. It was suddenly of utmost importance to me to complete the partially erased picture. I desperately wanted the answers to questions about the woman from my past. Did we work together? Did we get along? Did we argue? Were we friends or enemies? I was certain that she was unaware of my brain injury with amnesia, but I was too embarrassed to approach her with the information. My fear of supplying an enemy from the past with a weapon with which to harm me seemed cowardly to me later, and I was ashamed. Why is trust so difficult? Eventually, I learned that we worked together at a company where I was a long time cost accountant. But I still do not know anything about our relationship.

Pre-injury, I was a clever, strong, and efficient woman. I was also stern, and did not suffer fools gladly. During my professional life, I had many friends, because I enjoyed the comradeship of my associates. I was always part of any fun and laughter. However, my inflexible, business side made enemies for me. I regret that I did not have a less chiseled manner. What I will say in my defense is that I felt driven to acquire the respect of the many layers of management over me. That was a formidable task for an aging, undereducated female who lacked beauty. My strongest asset was my good brain.

Was this experience at the cookware party an example of short-term or long-term memory impairment? The ability to remember your home and family, long-time friends and neighbors, favorite music or movies, how to put on pants or brush your teeth are all considered long-term memory. More recent occurrences and acquaintances are usually considered short-term memory. I worked with this woman for a few years almost ten years ago. In what category does this kind of memory reside?

Found...

"Life is what happens to you while you're busy making other plans."
-John Lennon

Life with brain injury is a mystery adventure. Just when you have it figured out and you have settled into a sometimes challenging but manageable existence, a sudden plot twist throws you off balance.

Pain

You may wonder if there is pain with brain injury. Does it hurt? The answer is yes; then it becomes an annoying sensation, like a rash. I remember fierce, debilitating headaches, which interfered with my therapy. I wish that a more effective treatment was used when I was at Kernan. Pain is a vivid memory of my time there. A couple of months post injury; the pain subsided and left behind a sensation of wearing a too-tight hat. Since I was also recovering from assorted skull fractures, how did I categorize the sensations? I couldn't at first, but more than a year later, I divided it as follows: A) Pressure which seems to come from the outside (a too-tight hat or a rubber band around my head) is a healing scalp or skull. B) Pressure emanating from the inside (bugs or beetles running loose, electrical impulses, or a balloon sensation) is brain pain.

In the beginning, there can be intense discomfort. The pain of brain injury is a unique and debilitating headache. It is unlike a migraine, tension, or sinus headache, because it feels like millions of tiny, fast-moving creatures biting you on the inside. Relief can be hard to find, but it would be a bonus for the patient. Careful handling is required, especially if the patient is unable to adequately describe it. I know that I could not have found the words at the time. If you encountered me during the first few weeks of my recovery from TBI, you would have caught me pulling my hair, and digging at my scalp with my fingers. I was just trying to get at the scampering critters in my brain. It may also have been difficult to get me to pay attention to you, and to respond appropriately to verbal cues. The annoying creatures can block thought, and can even interfere with auditory comprehension. The sensation of wearing a too-tight hat persisted for over two years. Currently, I have bundles of electrical impulses. There is no actual pain, just an annoying itch that roams around the left side of my head, deep under my scalp. Since there is no appropriate medication, I have to remember to keep my hands off my scalp.

Post-traumatic Stress Disorder

The sight of on coming traffic can cause an electrical shock to snap in my brain, especially if one of the vehicles is too close to the center line. I feel as if time either stops or it moves in slow motion, because the agony seems to go on forever. Outwardly, I may whimper, groan, or squeal. In addition, I may cling to the passenger side ceiling, sun visor, dashboard, or door handle. All of this must somehow be coped with by Mike, who is driving. He has joked that riding with me is like riding with a lunatic or a kidnap victim. I have joked that I should ride blindfolded. A motion picture of this activity would be funny to look at, but the personal experience of PTSD is a chronic terror.

Cooper finds a place to hide during a thunderstorm. I don't blame her; I feel like crawling under the bed. Pre-injury I was fearless; thunderstorm watching from the front or the back porch was a pleasure. Now, when the lightening flashes and crackles, and when the thunder booms and rattles the windows, I feel like a cat in a room full of rocking chairs. Even the gathering of dark clouds and the increasing wind fills me with dread – as if a disaster is about to happen.

If harshness of any kind is close to me, I find it very hard to cope with. It can be in the form of raised voices, mean words, or anger between family members, neighbors, or strangers. My former stoicism has been replaced by hyper-sensitivity. The worst part is not how I feel, but how I might behave. Control can still be an issue for me. Even though I try very hard to maintain it, I sometimes feel like I'm holding back a locomotive. If I lose control, then I am likely to yell, scream, and cry. Afterwards, I feel remorse, shame, and embarrassment. If the emotional scene is severe enough, then it may take days for me to recover.

The explosive, metal-to-metal crunch of auto accidents is especially nerve-jarring to me. I tend to hold my breath and cover my face when I hear it. We live on a main road and tend to experience the noise a few times a year. Another sound from my motor vehicle accident that has a dramatic effect on me is the roar of a medevac helicopter. For me, the identity of that sound is unmistakable. I have asked my counselor how it is possible to have post-traumatic stress disorder in conjunction with amnesia. He has informed me that the senses can store memory, too. That must be the reason why the only memory I have from my birthday shortly after the accident is the flavor of coconut cake.

Survivors like me are not the only ones who may experience PTSD; our loved ones may, too. My husband and children are likely to be overly concerned when they cannot reach me by phone in a short period of time (less than one hour.) As a result, my husband has supplied me with a cell phone to have with me at all times. Mike has become somewhat over-protective because of his PTSD. When we are apart, he checks on me frequently, and he doesn't like me to drive. Mike's over-protectiveness can be a strain on our relationship. The catastrophic event of 10/3/00 is my family's 911. Since that day we have drawn closer together, and we are likely never to be far away from each other. Therefore, we experience the positive side of post-traumatic stress disorder.

Susceptibility

One of the most distressing aspects of my disability is a feeling of being under siege – always fighting to protect my self-esteem. The primary cause is the barrage of behavioral corrections I endure. Ever since I emerged from coma, it seems like I am constantly being corrected, redirected, and chastised. I don't remember being subject to so much correcting since I was a child, and every one else was an authority figure. I felt intimidated then and tended to turn inward, looking for self-identity, because too many people on the outside expressed disappointment in me. Repeating this portion of my development is humiliating.

I'm a woman over 50 years old who is frequently treated like a slow, disobedient child. The worst part is that my intellect is developed enough to acknowledge my need for occasional correcting. I sometimes wonder if it would have been easier on me to recover only 50% of my cognitive functions instead of 80 - 90%. Also, the individuals responsible for most of the redirection are kind, caring people who have my best interests at heart. So, how can I object? I don't. I keep my mouth shut and let my pride take a hit.

Feeling nervous about my behavior makes me awkward sometimes, and perhaps I seem unfriendly or aloof. Furthermore, apologizing is something that I do too much of, and I get very annoyed with myself. But what else can I do? The continuous focus on my behavior by me, by my loved ones, and by the professionals with whom I consult, exhausts me. I'm sure that it is yet another cause of the chronic depression that plagues me. Since I will have a brain injury for the rest of my life, I see no end to the cycle of being corrected and feeling embarrassed by it. Obviously, I must find a way to minimize the effect on my psyche that doesn't include becoming hard. I never want to return to being the fortress-like woman I was pre-injury.

Dimmer-switch

Another condition causes challenges, complications, even depression. I call it my dimmer-switch brain. Perhaps the lighting in your home has a device, which enables you to reduce the brightness without switching off the power. This is a convenient way to set the mood for peaceful dining, cozy conversation, or serene solitude. A more practical use is to conserve electricity. I am almost constantly aware of a personal impression of reduced brightness, close to dullness. I feel like someone used an emery board on all of my former sharpness. A suggestion to chill out is sometimes redundant, because brain injury can be built-in sedation. A dimmer-switch brain is both positively and negatively charged. The plus side is stress suppression; the negative side is a feeling of stupidity. I am definitely a tortoise surrounded by hares. I will eventually get to the finish line, but I may celebrate two birthdays along the way. However, savoring a slower existence can yield much pleasure.

Power Surge

Now my story takes an unexpected turn, because I have recently become aware of another cognitive phenomenon. I call it power surge. Post injury, whenever I have been presented with a situation requiring problem solving, speedy comprehension, or sound judgment, I have frequently been at a loss. Then, six months ago, I was attempting to work on a project, which I started and failed to finish a year ago – a table to help organize detailed information. My failure was due to lack of comprehension. However, as soon as I reviewed the project, I had a rush of clear, absolute understanding. I finished the project enthusiastically with hardly any difficulty. As I was still basking in this new light of power, the next project came along and proved to be too challenging for my injured brain – how to fit my dog's neck chain. Indeed, a portion of it was a stunning defeat. I immediately fell into that dark place of sadness where I don't like to be - a depression chamber. But then, another situation quickly followed that required improvisation to solve the problem of loss of detailed instructions – a hand-smocked garment. I had to create another way to achieve the same result. The solution occurred to me in a powerful surge of ideas. The one I chose worked perfectly, and I felt brilliant! A surge protector for my brain is the last thing I want. These stories illustrate that an injured brain can retain unexpected pockets of brilliance. The accelerated rate at which I relearned everything illuminated my life. I felt turned on - a little high. The CD player from my hospitalization resides in my kitchen, and is no longer a mystery to me. My thirst for knowledge about brain injury enabled me to acquire a better understanding of it, so it has become less scary.

Jell-O Molds and Spider

The brain is control-central for all of us. This incredibly complex computer that we never leave home without contains the essence of which we are, and enables us to interact with the rest of the world. Consider your computer at home or at your place of employment. You are aware that the hard case on the outside protects delicate parts on the inside. What would happen to it if you dropped it or a filing cabinet fell on it? Suppose your computer became infected with a dreaded virus, or that drops of water from a leaky ceiling got inside. Would you be concerned, angry, or devastated? The brain is a million times more sophisticated and delicate than your computer. Suppose you needed to transport a very special Jell-O mold to a party. What precautions would you take? If you dropped it when you got out of the car, what would happen to it? How would you feel? Except for color, there is a very strong resemblance between a brain and a Jell-O mold.

A very common creature is famous for building and maintaining a structure that can illustrate diffuse axonal brain injury -- the spider. It can quickly cover an area with a net made of very sensitive and delicate fibers. The thin threads are perfectly spaced in order to cover the pre-determined area most effectively. Signals travel instantly along this well-connected network to the owner, who can decode the messages and act accordingly. If a branch falls, tearing apart some of the connections, the determined spider can form new ones. The new structure may not exactly resemble the old, but it may function very well. The brain's axons can sometimes reach around damaged areas, finding and making new connections. This process is much slower than the spider's, though. It can take weeks, months, or years. In addition, the new connections may transfer thoughts, memories, or functions to areas not as skilled as the originals.

My neurologist, Dr. Michael Makley, has informed me that I very likely sustained a combination closed head injury. The left side of my brain took a direct hit when the pickup truck penetrated the driver's side of my car, possibly striking my head, causing blunt force trauma. Then, because my brain was set in motion within my skull, I acquired a diffuse axonal injury. The inside of our skulls is not smooth, because it actually has crags, points, and ridges, especially behind our faces. What would happen to your computer if you picked it up and shook it once or twice before setting it down again? Another major difference between the electronic device and the Jell-O mold in my skull is replacement parts. Computers have them; brains do not. However, I am very excited about stem-cell therapies for neural injury as presented by Dr. Vassilis Koliatsos at the annual BIAM conference. Imagine a way to repair the brain after an injury! We need to support stem cell research to keep the possibility alive.

Over the years, particular behaviors, attitudes, tastes, and mannerisms had become associated with me. When in certain situations, or when offered certain choices, I had become predictable. I would not say that such habitual behavior was boring, but it was definitely comfortable. When presented with a situation that requires participation in the form of developing questions or ideas, prioritizing, or problem solving, I now assume a position of passive observer. This requires that I focus on ignoring my former habit of taking a leadership position. Some advantages of the new habit are, less opportunity for my deficits to be exposed, and more time for processing and comprehending information.

If I have a list of any kind to remember, however small, my new habit is to journalize everything. More time is required, but reliance upon a phenomenal memory is no longer possible. Pockets, purses, surfaces, and spirals are being filled constantly, and therefore need cleaning out periodically. Unfortunately, if a family member asks for information from an old, discarded list, I am unlikely to have recall. But the use of lists and calendar notes frees me from having to try to remember so much.

Compensatory strategies can be developed by anyone to ease living with brain injury. For any project I undertake that has several steps to completion, my new habit is as follows: A) Divide and complete -- meaning, finish one part at a time, if possible. B) Plan, practice, and rehearse. Meaning, gather all the materials or ingredients, and line them up in order of use. Rehearse each step in your brain, until you are extremely familiar with the procedures. Keep written instructions in front of you, and put away each ingredient as you finish with it. My new habit means that I require more time than I used to, but it also allows me to be productive. *Extreme* organization is very handy to ease deficits in memory and for successful job completion.

In a circumstance where many tasks and jobs are waiting for someone to work on them, either at home or at the office where I volunteer, I am still trying to form new habits. I still catch myself reverting to old habitual behavior, which is trying to do it all myself. This can have devastating results because of extreme fatigue. My new and reduced stamina requires that I work on one task at a time before starting another. If I can only complete one job, then I must try to be satisfied with my accomplishment.

Formerly, pride drove me to try to over-achieve. It was an attempt to surround myself with an aura of importance. I assumed that doing more work than anyone did, and working longer hours than anyone, would make me indispensable to my employers. The actual truth was that I was fortunate if they remembered my name. The stress and fatigue generated by this old habit is no longer possible for me to cope with.

I am also embarrassed to admit that I wasted years looking for humanity in an environment where none exists – the business world. My new conviction that human compassion, caring, and concern are not present in private industry is an impediment to my seeking employment there. Instead, I made a home for myself at the Brain Injury Association of Maryland where humanity is the essence of their being. My boss, Diane Triplett, executive director, exhibited profound understanding of my disability. She accepted and welcomed me, as I am, not seeking to make changes, only to educate. I loved my job! How many can say that? Suzanne Kantt, assistant director, trustingly gave me a share in her projects, even patiently repeating instructions, if I forgot.

My experiences lead me to conclude that if one awakens to an unfamiliar self, then one should get to work immediately on self-knowledge. Find out what the new person iscapable of, and make full use of the strengths and talents discovered. Remember to change habits where necessary and to develop compensatory strategies in order to minimize challenges. Fulfillment and satisfaction at your job are still possible.

Eileen + Brain Injury = Rebirth

I have two birthdays - October 21, 1951 and October 3, 2000. It seems that I am destined to be a Libra, seeking balance, but living on a roller coaster. It is no wonder that I am jumpy and not relaxed. My first childhood was abusive, unhappy, and traumatizing. I tend not to look back on it fondly. My second childhood was bewildering, nurturing, and illuminating. I have a very strong preference for the second one.

Curiosity takes me back to my second childhood to revisit what is fascinating to me, but the experience can leave me shaken. It was a time of very high emotion, especially whenever I was without my security blanket, Mike. I still have a very strong desire to take the child, Eileen, in my arms, dry her tears, and rock her gently. She was just scared, because she did not understand anything. She felt like everyone was picking on her, telling her what to do, what not to do, and sometimes even hurting her. Everything was under their control - getting up, eating, therapy, bathroom breaks, and going to bed. Nothing was fun and she did not like anyone; they all just made her mad. Life was so unfair! If doctors, nurses, therapists, and technicians could see inside an injured brain, they would find a quivering, half-starved puppy with a hurt paw. For that puppy to thrive and learn to trust, it takes tenderness, patience, love, and nurturing.

The gentler moments happened when a staff member was especially careful and considerate. That helped me to relax and be less angry. The quivering puppy with a hurt paw feeling persisted rather strongly for two to three years, through most of my surgeries. My husband is still the best at comforting me.

Every October 3, I not only wish myself a happy birthday, but I also divide my life into two parts, called pre-injury and post-injury. I think that I will always admire the pre-injury adult for several reasons. I was a bright, highly motivated, over-achiever type, and my employers were glad to have me. Learning new skills, problem-solving, and multi-tasking came naturally. I was also a good wife and mother. As a post-injury adult, I get more satisfaction from life, because I am more accessible - very different from the fortress-like woman of the past. I am also much more fearful, and I experience more failures, but my successes are inspirational. Being more expressive makes me a better wife, I think. Mike and I are closer than ever, and our love is even stronger. However, I have genuine concerns about my parenting skills post-injury. Since I believe that good parents are *strong and effective* individuals, I am probably disqualified. My adult children sometimes reveal their disappointment in my new persona. The families of persons with brain injury must come to terms with it, too.

Our granddaughter, Lucy Eileen Matson, was born on February 13, 2004, and she is the best thing that ever happened to this family. She is the ray of sunshine that we all needed after more than three dark years following my brain injury. Lucy doesn't know that her Nana is disabled. She has only known me as I am now. Therefore, she has no regrets associated with our relationship. I feel at ease with Lucy, because she doesn't mind if I'm a little slow, or if I can't find the words. Indeed, as she grows, she tends to help me almost as much as I help her. Our granddaughter teaches all of us how to get the most out of life. She doesn't worry about the small things that can go wrong. She just moves on to the next activity if it does. Lucy is a highly intelligent and happy child, and I love to hear her laugh.

I am happy to report that we have acquired another dog from the ASPCA. She was rescued at six weeks old from the streets of Baltimore. She is a medium to large lab/chow mix, the color of a deer, with appealing brown eyes. Cooper II is a people-loving dog who has made many friends in the neighborhood. We love her very much.

To contemplate my recovery thus far is gratifying. God's blessings for me are in the souls of other people, and the names of some of the individuals are in this book. During my "quiet times", He has also reminded me of my own determination. I still have strong disagreements with Him, but I am mostly at peace. However mysterious His plan is, I am glad to still be part of it.

The following is a summary of what I have found to date, post-injury.

- Love - the ability to feel it more deeply, to express it more openly, to gather a larger quantity, and to spread it more widely.

- Adventure - to find it in ordinary days, to anticipate it when I wake up, and to let it be a source of happiness.

- Laughter - learning to be my own greatest source of amusement, to let it out, and to catch it from others.

- Spirituality - to feel childlike, to let inspiration penetrate my soul, to be close enough to God to get mad at Him, to be quiet and let Him speak.

- Sensuality - to be excited by colors, tastes, sounds, scents, and my skin, to more fully enjoy sexual gratification.

- Gratitude - to believe that to be beholden to someone is good, because it is evidence of caring that we can never have or do enough of.

- Life - ceasing to squander the moments, slowing down enough to revel in it, and recognizing the gift of it all around me.

- People - to enjoy the variety, companionship, inspiration, and mutual aid.

- Wisdom - discovering that the more I give, the more I receive. Looking for and finding my hidden pockets of intelligence, while discarding old baggage.

- Freedom - psychological closet cleaning and reorganizing - out with the bad, in with the good.

- Peace - concluding that I am okay. Acceptance

- Humility – to enjoy the serenity of it, to be satisfied just to be, to surrender my soul.

- Motivation – to enjoy the feeling of inner strength, to feel confident, to rejoice in the successful results.

- Pain – sometimes physical, sometimes psychological.

- PTSD – something I can share with my family.

- Susceptibility – looking for a way to protect myself.

I wrote the following poem more than 25 years ago. Then, I revised it in 2004 for inclusion in the newsletter, <u>Headstand</u>, which BIAM used to have printed. The words have more significance to me now.

A Gift

Merely a marigold, my voice is small,
but my life's the greatest lesson of all.
Waiting behind the flower I give
is a seed that says I must die to live.
Thrilled at your pleasure 'cause my colors are bold,

I laughingly reflect the sun's own gold.
As you weed and water and care for me,
I am satisfied just to be.

But, your smile fades away
when you find that I cannot stay.
"Oh God," you say. "What have I done?"
You thought our time had just begun.

Don't grieve my friend 'cause you feel forlorn.
Now is the time for which I was born.
When, in your stark and wintry despair,
you breathe the scent of springish air,
search among the leaves of old,
and find the offspring of the marigold.

School Days...

"There's nothing you can know that isn't known, nothing you can see that isn't shown, nowhere you can be that isn't where you're meant to be. It's easy. All you need is love."
-The Beatles

Within the core of me lived a fervent wish, lying dormant through the decades, until the time was right for it to be free. My early life was spent in a household where my father decreed that girls were not worth educating. Then, at the age of nineteen, I married, and my husband and I became the parents of two children by the time we were twenty-five years old. During the decades following these events, I devoted all my energy and resources to being a good wife and mother. Eventually, I began a career in accounting – starting at the bottom. There was never time, money, or opportunity together simultaneously, for me to pursue my education, until the life changing event of Y2K.

The steps leading to my first moments as a college student included the "people helping people" factor – formerly unused and unappreciated by me. Pre-injury, I was a stoic, fortress of a woman. Whenever I was presented with a particularly difficult problem in my profession, I worked hard (in my cubicle) looking for a solution – occasionally consulting with the resident experts. I was a loner; working late hours and on weekends was my preference. They say that pride leads to a fall. My prideful habit cost me a good brain.

By the winter of 2007, I was ready for a change. The four years spent volunteering with the Brain Injury Association of Maryland greatly rehabilitated my thinking and honed my administrative skills, but it was time for the next step. I was ready to take the sage advice from the early days with my professional counselor. Dr. Hopkins had said, "Why don't you take some classes at Carroll Community College?" At the time that he suggested it, I strongly rejected the idea. I was still deeply depressed and disengaged from life. Five years later, I was ready to listen – but the enthusiasm of my husband, Mike, was the clincher.

Carroll Community College in Westminster, Maryland welcomes serious students from every conceivable source – a common interest of many learning institutions. The college has a designated advisor for students with disability, and my first meeting with her was a revelation. It was her job to make sure that I started my college career without unreasonable expectations, and I left her office feeling more disabled than when I entered. All the information presented to me seemed massive in quantity and cryptically inaccessible. The heart that I had set on going to school was breaking, until the thing in me that had not been killed in the accident came to my rescue. With determination, I set about gathering transcripts, filling out forms, visiting the local Social Security office (for the tuition waiver), and taking the placement exams. Starting at the beginning seemed like excellent advice, so I enrolled in English 101 and became a student. The college offers reasonable accommodations to students like me, and I recommend that anyone with a disability and a desire to be a college student takes advantage of what is offered.

The two accommodations that I use the most are: Extra time

to complete quizzes and tests, and the option to take tests and exams in the testing center. The testing center ensures that there will be absolutely no distractions for someone like me. Today, I am great friends with the specialist for students with disability, Joyce Sebian. I treasure her learned advice and encouraging support. She has lifted my spirits with kind expressions of her pride in my accomplishments. With the help of Mike, Dr. Hopkins, and Joyce

Sebian, I am succeeding as a student. I am happily experiencing a life-long wish.

On that first evening in May 2007, I took a deep breath and walked under a sign that read, "Enter to Learn." When the doors slid open, an invigorating aroma of books, paper, and people wrapped itself around me, and I entered eagerly – my book bag slung over my shoulder. I was an aging female with a traumatic brain injury, who had not been in school for thirty-seven years, and I was scared. Carroll Community College is a fairly new, well-kept, and beautiful campus. Over the past fifteen years, buildings have been built around the original rectangular two-story structure, some at an angle, but connected with breezeways. There are eight red brick buildings with cobalt blue roofs, and one amphitheater. My classroom was in the basement of one of the side attachments. I entered and chose a seat in the front – the better to absorb everything. Twenty more students wandered in silently and scattered like tumbleweeds around the room. We were a mixed mass of male and female, old and young, and eager and listless. A diminutive woman, about ten years my junior, entered last, trailing a heavy-looking bag on wheels. In a soothing and kindly manner, she introduced herself as our English instructor, and the odyssey commenced. I was immediately drawn to her warm, relaxed manner. During our time together, I learned that to possess an aptitude for writing is not sufficient by itself. I also needed to pay attention to the details of my writing so that my expressions were clear and mostly error free. Her sincere appreciation of my work was always refreshing and inspired me to work toward self-improvement. Joann Pilachowski and I have formed a close personal relationship since I left her classroom.

My English 102 professor was energetically enthusiastic. She made reading short stories, poetry, and drama adventurous. With her, I learned to analyze what I was reading, to ponder themes, and to notice symbolism. In addition, I learned to write concisely and to say what I mean. She was also positively impressed with my writing, and I was thrilled. I have used the lessons from both of my English professors to improve this book, and Suzanne Dixon has also become a friend.

For both Art Appreciation and Introduction to Film, my instructor was a kind-hearted young artist. She stirred my interest in art forms and in artists, beyond my old favorites, and I learned how to harness my impressions into organized critical thinking. Now I view motion pictures with an eye for editing techniques and mise-en-scene (the physical setting of an action.) Stephanie Halpern and I formed a relationship that is simpatico.

One of the most challenging and interesting courses I have taken so far is Anthropology. My professor was extremely knowledgeable about different cultures, but her sense of fun and imaginative lesson plans made the challenging course work easier to learn. Mel Hall used props to teach us about different cultures, including costumes, which she would remove in class and discuss the origin and significance of each piece. She also brought her guitar to class for a sing-along of old folk music from different eras and regions.

Next, Sociology was made easier because of its relationship to Anthropology. My Sociology instructor, Gail Spessert, listened patiently to our opinions with an unbiased manner. She, like Mel Hall, provided creative lesson plans that included group activities, which are an excellent resource for survivors of brain injury to relearn social skills.

My History professor, Ray D'Amario, was a man about ten years my senior and so knowledgeable about the material, that it was incredible. For my History class and everything that came before, I needed to create some compensatory strategies to help me remember a huge amount of facts, dates, people, and places. Therefore, I created tables either by hand or on Microsoft Word. In addition, the color-coding of related subject matter has been extremely useful – different colors of highlighters on white paper or colored paper for printing. Since my memory is more visual than it used to be, I made tables that were organized by date (like time lines) on different subjects such as, authors and their works, The Age of Enlightenment, and The First World War. If I studied these tables, I found that I could picture them later for test taking. The strategies worked very well. Here is an example of a table for English class; this was printed on pink (for poetry) paper:

Title	Author	Year	Notes
Death be not Proud	John Donne	1610	Because of eternal life, death will die Paradox
To the Virgins, to Make Much of Time	Robert Herrick	1648	Carpe Diem - seize the day - "gather ye rosebuds while ye may"
Wild Nights - Wild Nights	Emily Dickenson	18861	Secret lover: year of her mental breakdown
"Out, Out -"	Robert Frost	1916	Allusion -Macbeth; 16-year-old boy cuts off hand with malfunctioning saw
Harlem (Dream Deferred)	Langston Hughes	1951	Simile that ends with metaphor; series of questions with dramatic end
Do not go gentle into that good night	Dylan Thomas	1952	Poem to his father - don't die without a fight

Another strategy that has worked well for me for writing papers is the use of index cards. The points I wanted to make in my paper were noted on the cards, along with the identity of the source from which the information was taken. Then, I applied a color-coding label over the top of the card that matched the label on the photocopied resource. I wrote a paper about the effect of depression on three famous people, Edgar Allan Poe, Brian Wilson, and Hunter S. Thompson, using this method. The paper was well received by my instructor, and illustrated that organization is a key that enables successful completion of assignments.

Have you ever used an acronym? I bet you have. It is a word

made up of the first letters of a list of words in order to better remember the list. Here is an acronym I used for Art Appreciation class to help me remember the Seven Principles of Design:

BRECUDS

1. B – Balance
2. R – Repetition and Rhythm
3. E – Emphasis and Subordination
4. C – Contrast
5. U – Unity and Variety
6. D – Directional Forces
7. S – Scale and Proportion

Around the corner, however, there lurked a significant obstacle to my goal of obtaining a college degree. I had acquired a serious math deficit due to my brain injury – an overwhelming humiliation for a former accountant. One of the results of taking the college placement exams was the discovery of this deficit. Joyce Sebian devised a plan to both ease the humiliation and to help me overcome the hurdle. She lent me instructor text books on math (with answers in the back) to study, and suggested that I take a non-credit math-prep course. All of this was to prepare me to re-take the math placement exam. Until I succeeded in scoring higher on the exam, I was not qualified to earn the credits I needed in Biology, Science, and Math toward my degree. After approximately one year of self-study, I went to the testing center at the college one morning. Two hours later, I emerged shaken, but triumphant. I managed to score *two* levels higher in math! I had qualified to take a credit math course – the gate-keeper to the math/science portion of my degree! No one was more proud of me than my husband, but both Dr. Hopkins and Joyce Sebian ran a close second.

It was one thing to proudly register for the hard-earned math course, and quite another to sit in class with quick-minded youngsters and not make a fool of myself. During the months of self-study I filled spirals with algebra problems. Since this method worked well for me, I decided to use it for class. I quickly filled another spiral with practice problems and I was only halfway through the semester! Every day I copied problems from my textbook and labored to find the solutions. An online website, www.Mathxl.com, was also a big help for practice. Soon, my test grades demonstrated that I was not wasting my time. The in-class lectures proved to be another hurdle for me to overcome. What could I do? Because of my slower processing speed, I needed a strategy to help me avoid being left far behind by the lectures; so I developed a very simple one. Using the instructor's syllabus, I worked one day ahead of the lecture – even doing practice problems. This enabled me to both ask intelligent questions in class and to also answer questions intelligently.

Distractibility is a common side-effect of brain injury. This most annoying aspect of me is what could have led to my ultimate failure in math. My first few experiences in math lab left me desperate and depressed. The atmosphere was crowded, noisy, and hot (because of the computers.) In addition, the instructor traveled around the room, leaning over the students' shoulders to both peer at and to correct their work. This completely unnerved me and rendered me incapable of focusing or thinking. Furthermore, since I was working math problems on a website instead of with pencil and paper, I had to learn to use the new tools (on the computer) at the same time that I was recalling and utilizing math concepts. A consultation with Joyce Sebian yielded a solution. The large math lab contained a number of infrequently used wooden cubicles with computers. I obtained permission to take math lab in a cubicle, and in addition, my instructor graciously agreed to not approach me unless I signaled for her help. The strategy worked; my lab gradesimproved dramatically. Is it not incredible to consider that such a small change can make the world of difference to someone like me?

Failure to make the best use of time can also be an unwelcome intruder in the life of a brain injury survivor. We can become obsessed with one detail of a larger picture while time disappears. Unfortunately, this circumstance happened when I was taking a math test. I am ashamed to admit that I spent, perhaps, twelve minutes on one problem that baffled me. When I remembered to look at the clock, I was horrified to have squandered so much time. I rushed to finish the test, which is another hazard for people like me. When we are stressed, pressured, or rushed, our thinking abilities are diminished. My score on that test was well below the two previous ones, and I was also humiliated to note that most of my errors were simple addition or subtraction. I needed another strategy. Therefore, on future tests, I noted the total number of questions first, then I divided that number into the total amount of time I had for the exam. The resulting number was how many minutes I could afford to spend on each problem, but I had to be disciplined. In addition, I was able to set goals during the test such as, the number of questions that must be completed by the end of the first hour. My test scores proved that the plan worked. My math professor, Larry Schlude, was very patient and supportive. Without his cooperation, I would not have been able to successfully face down my challenges.

Speech class was a sometimes painful educational experience – like exposure therapy. My professor was a PhD and a performance skills expert. He taught us to overcome our public speaking anxieties by doing. We researched, wrote, rehearsed, and presented speeches in class, followed by classmate critiques, followed by instructor critiques. We had all grown very thick skins by the time we gave our last speeches. I learned that even a well-written speech can be obscured by a poor performance. I am grateful to Dr. Darren Goins for the experience, and I am sure that the lessons learned will improve my public speaking.

Here is something else I learned in speech class – memory skills practice. First, make a list of items, numbered one to ten. Then, draw a picture beside each item that represents both the number and the item.

1. Foot – draw one foot.
2. Chair – draw two chairs
3. Pin – draw three pins
4. Tree – draw a tree with four branches
5. Pie – draw a round pie, cut into five portions
6. Ladder – draw a ladder with six rungs
7. Snake – draw a serpent with a forked tongue in the shape of a number seven
8. Spider – draw an eight-legged bug

9. Clock – draw a round clock with the hands at nine o'clock
10. Lace – draw five pairs of eyelets with a shoelace crisscrossed through them

Next, take a minute to look at the list before covering it. Finally, try to recite the list out loud. I was surprised at how much easier it was to remember the list because I could picture it. Perhaps you will have the same experience.

Phi Theta Kappa

When a survivor of severe TBI qualifies for induction into Phi Theta Kappa, the international honor society for two-year colleges, what can be said? With the humanbrain, anything is possible is, perhaps, an appropriate conclusion. Just over eight years ago after emerging from coma, I was struggling to relearn everything that an infant is taught. Now I have received a letter of congratulations and invitation from the college president to join a prestigious society. On the evening of the induction I was very pleased to have my family present as well as Joyce Sebian, Dr. Bill Hopkins, and my English 102 professor, Suzanne Dixon. On stage with the rest of the executive board, I even had a small speaking role before presenting a white rose to each of the one hundred inductees. My heart was beating fast and my cheeks were bright red, but, except for the few roses that I knocked off the table to the stage floor, everything went well. As we gathered on the grand staircase for a group picture, I touched the small gold emblem pinned to my sweater and realized something very important. I had reached another level in my recovery. Furthermore, something outside of my disability was being celebrated – recognition of my *ability*. More importantly, I belonged to a larger society.

At home, my dear Mike paid me the greatest compliment. He is a great fan of Sir Arthur Conan Doyle's Sherlock Holmes, and knows all of the adventures. He quoted from the final paragraphs of <u>The Adventure of the Six Napoleons</u>. Inspector Lestrade, who is usually at odds with Holmes, says, "…We're not jealous of you at Scotland Yard. No, sir, we are very proud of you, and if you come down tomorrow, there's not a man, from the oldest inspector to the youngest constable, who wouldn't be glad to shake you by the hand." I was deeply moved because I know how much Mike admires the cleverness of Sherlock Holmes.

I have started another semester at Carroll Community College, and I have a strong desire to share some of my study strategies with my classmates, so I am training to be a peer tutor. Experience and greater confidence will be useful tools for this endeavor.

The benefits of going to college are the same for brain injury survivors as they are for anyone else. But, one could argue that there is more urgency for survivors to become college students because of the need for cognitive rehabilitation. I have advocated for the college experience with my support group because of the following personal benefits:

- Knowledge

- Thinking fitness

- Problem solving skills

- Interpersonal skills (socialization, self-esteem, self-confidence)

Knowledge

Acquiring knowledge is not only the act of filling one's head with facts and details, but also the act of broadening one's perspective. Learning about the where, the what, and the why of humanity in Anthropology and in Sociology, was invaluable. Once upon a time, I understood Eileen very well. I knew her beliefs, her preferences, her habits, her strengths, and her weaknesses. She was lost in that car wreck all those years ago. She has been replaced by a new person who was still in the process of being discovered. Studying the convictions and the resulting patterns of behavior of humanity over time and worldwide has cleared my brain of worthless bias, preconceptions, and stereotypes. Therefore, understanding me has been made easier through understanding others. Studying history reveals where we have been, what we did, and what the results were. This knowledge *should* improve our decision making skills, and heaven knows that having good decision making skills can be especially challenging for survivors of brain injury. Sometimes I look at current world leaders and wonder if they have BI in their histories. The follies and misunderstandings that have led human beings into conflict with each other through the centuries are exposed in history. Can we not take valuable lessons from the past to help us live more successfully now and in the future? Studying the creative drive in ancient humans and in people of today reveals a very important fact; we have not changed that much. We still share a life with each other that some of us feel compelled to decorate. Learning that I have so much in common with the rest of humanity can ease the painful self perception of being different. More importantly, learning about something new is about discovering possibilities, which is where hope lies.

Thinking fitness

Thinking fitness is about exercise. If you fail to exercise your body, then you will lose muscle mass, making your body a less than reliable tool with which to navigate through life. Exercising your brain can actually increase its connectivity. The more connections you have and the stronger they are, the sharper your thinking. In addition, exercising the brain increases its ability to withstand and to recover from disease and trauma. Many BI survivors have slower processing speeds. I am no different. Consider this: studying is thinking, the more I study, the more thinking practice I have, and the more I practice thinking, the more skilled at it I become. I took that lesson from the great Brooks Robinson of the Baltimore Orioles. He was not born a superb third baseman, but he practiced and honed his skills for decades, including on the last day that he played professional baseball in 1977. He exemplifies the possibilities if you just practice.

Problem solving

People like me need to improve our problem solving skills, and successful college students develop sound problem solving skills. Every day we spend time prioritizing, organizing our day's activities according to what needs to be accomplished and when. Obstacles that can prevent us from completing assignments are inevitable. Lack of comprehension of the instructions or material, technology failure, and research dead ends are some of the possibilities. But finding ways to surmount the obstacles is problem solving practice. I have experienced all of the above and more, and my advice is as follows: don't try to do it alone; get someone to help you. If you do not understand an assignment, get clarification from your instructor. He or she is happy to answer questions, if the result is successful completion of the assignment. If you cannot reach your professor, or if you still have difficulty understanding, get a loved one, a friend, or a classmate to explain their understanding. If your computer fails at home, get on the phone to a help line, or get a loved one to help you. If your home computer is unreliable, make time to work on assignments at school, where the technology is more reliable and paid staff is available to help you. If you reach a dead end while researching a written assignment, ask the library staff if they can help you. One of the duties of the college library staff is to help students with research; they are trained for it.

Interpersonal skills

A very important step in human development is socialization. It is essential for all of us to learn how to interact with other people, since we share this life with each other. Community college contains an assortment of students from every classification – young, old, rich, poor, male, female, career oriented, family oriented, and different ethnicities. We learn to work together to complete assignments in diverse groups, large and small. As we do this, we practice interpersonal skills. Isolation, often self-imposed, can hamper the redevelopment of a person post-injury. My own perception of feeling different from and therefore, separate from the rest of humanity has been challenged by interacting with my classmates. Since we have no choice but to engage in shared activities like, sitting next to one another for five to fifteen weeks at a time, engaging in group discussions, and working on assigned group projects, we have to learn tolerance, respect, and reliability. I have discovered that the majority of my classmates have a certain amount of reluctance to interact with strangers; I am not alone. Furthermore, if I reach out to my classmates with a friendly word or smile, they almost always respond the same way. How can anyone avoid feeling encouraged and cheered by this activity? Faculty and staff also respond positively to my friendly attitude. They greet me with a nod and a smile when I encounter them in the hallways. Self-esteem is: loving yourself. To like other people, to show deference to others, and to display friendliness to others increases love of self. There are plenty of opportunities for this pleasant sensation every day at school.

A cousin of self-esteem is self-confidence. If you have the first, it is easier to possess the second. Belief in you is what self-confidence is all about. If you are facing a test or exam in a challenging subject, and you know that you have done all the work and have studied hard, then you have already fulfilled your duties as a student. Give yourself a pep-talk on the way to the exam, instead of thinking negatively. Remind yourself that you are a good student who is bound to do well on the test. If you earn a better than expected grade, then celebrate your achievement. Remember that you couldn't have done it without you.

I have mentioned my friend and mentor, Joyce Sebian, in this chapter. She was generous enough to lend me some more of her precious time by giving me this quote to share with you:

I met Eileen in March 2007 and became involved with her preparation to enter postsecondary education. From the onset, Eileen was determined and very motivated. She accepts that she has a disability and more than likely, in most cases, she will have to work harder than her peers. This has never been a deterrent for Eileen.

We discussed the possibility that she may have to take some transitional courses, particularly in Math, (an academic skill that was most impacted by TBI). Eileen expressed her desire to place into college level courses only and we worked on a plan that included the goal of assessment results at the college level. Eileen worked hard, studied long, and placed into a college level Math. We were both very happy.

Eileen is very judicious in everything she tackles; she will find ways to overcome any negatives that she encounters; she is a great self-advocate-soft-spoken, yet firm when she is sure of what she needs. When unsure or seeking affirmation, she is always open to suggestions, open to trying new approaches, and is not above having to do something more than once. Eileen does not recognize failure, just the need for a different approach to the concern.

Eileen's decision to share her story with others will be a wonderful catharsis for her and inspirational for everyone who reads it.

Joyce Sebian
Disability Support Services
Carroll Community College

Glasgow and Rancho...

The **Glasgow Coma Scale (GCS)** is based on a fifteen-point scale for estimating and categorizing the outcomes of brain injury based on overall social capability or dependence on others. The test measures the motor response, verbal response and eye opening response with the following values:

I. Motor Response

6 - Obeys commands fully

5 - Localizes to noxious (Pain) stimuli

4 - Withdraws from noxious (Pain) stimuli

3 - Abnormal flexion, I.e. decorticate posturing

2 - Extensor response, I.e. decerebrate posturing

1 - No response

II. Verbal Response

5 - Alert and Oriented

4 - Confused, yet coherent speech

3 - Inappropriate words and jumbled phrases consisting of words

2 - Incomprehensible sounds

1 - No sounds

III. Eye Opening

4 - Spontaneous eye opening

3 - Eyes open to speech

2 - Eyes open to pain

1 - No eye opening

The final score is determined by adding the values of **I + II + III**. This number helps medical practitioners categorize the four possible levels for survival, with a lower number indicating a more severe injury and a poorer prognosis.

Mild (13 - 15)

Moderate Disability (9 - 12)
- Loss of consciousness greater than thirty minutes
- Physical or cognitive impairments which may resolve
- Benefit from rehabilitation

Severe Disability (3 - 8)
- Coma: Unconscious state. No meaningful response; no voluntary activities.

Vegetative State (< 3)
- Sleep wake cycles
- Arousal, but no interaction with environment
- No localized response to pain

Persistent Vegetative State
- Vegetative state lasting longer than one month

The EMS team captain, Sam Mann, gave me a score of 5 at the scene – **I. Motor Response** *2 (extensor response),* **II. Verbal Response** *2 (Incomprehensible sounds),* **III. Eye Opening** *1 (No eye opening). At Shock Trauma, Dr. Cooper recorded a score of 8 or 9 in my record. That score was reduced to a 6 during*

*the first few days after the accident, but that was
in conjunction with heavy sedation. Therefore, my
degree of brain injury is moderate to severe.*

The **Rancho Los Amigos Scale** was developed at a California hospital as a convenient and universal means of describing a person's progression from deep coma to appropriate cognitive functioning and behavior. *When I obtained a score of 3 to 5 on this scale, I was transferred to Kernan, but my brain was still not recording memory.*

Level I: No Response. The patient is unconscious/appears to be sleeping. Does not respond to any stimuli.

Level II: Generalized Response. Patient reacts inconsistently and without purpose. Often gross body movement or garbled vocalization is the same regardless of stimuli. First response is usually from deep pain.

Level III: Localized Response. Patient is improving. Will react more specifically, but inconsistently to the type of stimulus presented. May occasionally follow simple commands.

Level IV: Confused-Agitated. Patient is very active, but severely confused and disoriented. Not yet able to understand what is going on. May exhibit bizarre behavior. May be hostile and uncooperative because of internal confusion. May perform automatic motor activities like sitting, reaching, and walking in an agitated state, but not as a purposeful act.

Level V: Confused-Inappropriate. Patient is less agitated. Can respond to simple commands more consistently. Commands that are more complex produce responses that are confused, non-purposeful and random. Agitated behavior is due to environment. Highly distractible and has difficulty learning new information. Memory is severely impaired. Can "wander off" the unit and verbalization is often inappropriate.

Level VI: Confused-Appropriate. Patient is motivated and shows goal-directed behavior. Still depends upon others to lead the way, and needs constant cueing. Old memory has greatly improved, but new memory is still impaired. Has more awareness of self and family. Can recognize staff members. Reactions are more appropriate.

Level VII: Automatic-Appropriate. Patient now oriented to person, place and time. Can do daily routines automatically, but is robot-like. Needs some supervision because of impaired judgment, problem-solving, and planning skills. Has awareness of, but no insight to, his/her condition.

Level VIII: Purposeful-Appropriate. Patient can integrate the past with recent events. Is independent and can function in society. There may be deficits in stress tolerance, judgment, abstract reasoning, processing information, and emotional capacities.

Level IX: Purposeful, Appropriate, Self-Monitoring. Correct responses; carryover of new learning. Assistance is required to identify and avoid problems before they occur. Low frustration tolerance.

Level X. Purposeful, Appropriate, Independent. Correct responses; accurately estimates abilities and independently adjusts to task demands. May exhibit periods of depression, irritability, and low frustration tolerance when under physiologic, physical, or emotional stress.

*My suggestions and experiences are in italics.

Levels I and II:

1. Talk to your loved one in normal conversational tones. Your relative may be able to hear more than you realize. Try playing your loved ones favorite music or taped messages from family and friends. *At this stage, Mike provided a small CD player and The Beatles CD's. Their music has been a part of me for over 40 years. Mike always made sure that The Beatles were heard by my bedside whenever he was there. He also told me that the hospital staff remembered to keep the CD's playing, so that it*

became an audible expectation of anyone entering or passing by my room.

He also placed in my arms a small, soft, pink, bear, and I became very attached to my little companion. Mike tells me that he witnessed my reported agitation when the bear was misplaced. My good arm continued to reach and search endlessly until my little friend was back in my arms.

I still have the little bear. Sometimes I hold it, stroking its soft fur, trying to imagine what it was like during the "big blank." The little one's wide-open eyes saw everything, but it cannot convey anything - except the strong love and devotion with which it arrived.

It is unknown how much a comatose person can hear or remember. Mike certainly held my hand to comfort me; perhaps he said, "Your pain won't last forever. You'll be okay. Don't give up." I remember that one of my earliest quests was to find the owner of this very kind voice who whispered in my ear. Even now, Mike neither claims ownership of the voice, nor does he deny it. He has told me that perhaps it was the voice of God. I strongly suspect that it was Mike's voice in my ear, because it was very familiar.

2. Inform the staff of your loved ones interests, because they often respond best to a favorite song or television show. *Mike told me that the hospital staff remembered to keep the CD player going in my room.*

3. This is the hardest time for the family. What you do may appear to have no effect, and this stage can go on for several months. *I was not able to stay awake for more than 5 minutes at a time.*

4. Provide stimulation for ten to fifteen minute intervals, but do not expect responses to everything. *At this stage, my family told me that I would tire very easily and would even fall asleep while they were speaking..*

Level III:

It is likely that I was transferred to Kernan at this point – still, I have no memory.

1. Be alert to any changes in your loved one's reaction to you. Since some persons respond best to familiar voices, you may be the first to notice a change. These must be reported to staff immediately. *Mike has told me that I always responded to him even when I didn't respond to anyone else.*

2. Continue to talk to the person in a normal conversational tone. *My sister told me that hospital staff would speak loudly into my ear to get a response. I would usually startle awake and then go right back to sleep. She thought they were too harsh.*

3. Give your loved one simple, one-step commands, like: "Squeeze my hand."

4. Allow <u>ample</u> reaction time before repeating instructions.

5. Do not continually question your relative to see "how they are doing." You may cause confusion, since it is unlikely that they recall recent events.

6. Provide frequent orientation to day of the week, time, place, and reason for their hospitalization; always use person's familiar name. Remind staff if they use an incorrect name. Repetition is important, since they will not remember your earlier explanation. Try crossing the days off a large calendar within their view. *Our son, Mike, always reminded me what day it was, according to my husband. I have no memory of this. Mike provided a sign, "Call me Eileen," for over my bed. The staff continually called me by my first name, Grace, even though I am known by my middle name. I still feel very uncomfortable when current health care providers call me Grace. It seems contradictory to have strangers, who do not know my name, examine my body or remind me of my next appointment.*

7. Allow the person adequate rest time. Intersperse activities and talking with rest periods. *Beth always made sure that I was bathed and tucked into bed during the evening visit.*

8. Frequently reassure your loved one that their needs are being met and that they are safe.

Level IV:

My first memory post-injury may have happened at this stage (being dressed in strange clothing for a doctor's appointment, an uncomfortable ride in the back of a van). It was also at this time that my 29th wedding anniversary occurred; sadly, I don't remember anything about it.

1. Provide a calm, soothing, relaxed atmosphere during visits. If you get upset or angry, leave the room and return when you regain your composure.

My sisters are still resentful of a nurse at Shock Trauma they refer to as "sarge." They had been strongly chided for becoming hysterical in my presence. I am sure that my condition was hard for them to look at, and recovery must have seemed impossible. However, this is an example of the nurse-to-patient dedication that is so important for good recovery. I am very grateful to have had excellent patient-focused care.

2. Use short, simple directions and repeat them frequently.

3. Simplify your vocabulary and slow down your rate of speech. Be careful not to talk to your loved one like a child.

4. Do not expect the person to remember recent events or instructions. Tell the person what you

want them to know. If you quiz him or her, this will increase irritability.

5. Help your loved one to stay oriented to date, hospital, city, and cause of hospitalization by providing the facts. It is okay to correct the person gently, but do not argue or criticize them for forgetfulness.

Mike had to correct my younger sister more than once about ceasing to remind me about our childhood. It was probably her way of coping with the horror of watching me attempt to emerge from coma. Thank God that Mike understood how important it was to keep me oriented to the present. It must have been disturbing for him to witness my continued lapses into childhood, which was not good for me.

6. If restraints are being used, leave them in place. They are present for the person's security, protection, and safety during the time of disorientation and agitation.

Level V:

My birthday may have happened at this point, but all I can remember is the flavor of coconut cake. Mike says that I ate too much cake and ice cream and became ill.

1. Provide cues, which will enable your loved one to automatically answer your questions about past or

current events correctly.

Example: "Didn't you meet your wife in high school?" instead of "Where did you meet your wife?"

2. Supply fewer reminders to complete tasks. Your loved one should now be able to focus and remember for two to three minutes at a time.

3. Continue to use simple vocabulary and directions, but do not treat the person like a child.

4. Correct inaccurate statements gently.

5. If your loved one becomes upset, change the

topic, give them a brief rest period, or calmly suggest that they relax.

6. Avoid open-ended questions. Example: "What did you have for breakfast?" or "Do you know where you are?" Provide the information. *My family was constantly telling me about current events (The World Series, Presidential Election.)*

Level VI:

At this stage, I was likely in the last week to ten days at Kernan. I also have a larger collection of memories from this time, including reading The Beatles Anthology. Mike tells me that it was a present from him for my birthday.

1. Use normal conversation, but be specific. He or she will not "get" involved jokes or sarcasm.

2. Your loved one should now be able to work with you on tasks for ten to fifteen minutes.

3. The person may be able to answer questions about their past, their treatment schedule, or very recent important events without cues.

4. Help your loved one to journalize their daily activities, and review the list with them. *Mike helped me to write down my list of therapies for the current day and for the next day.*

5. Keep your loved one motivated to participate in all their therapies. They may refuse, because they do not acknowledge their limitations.

Level VII:

This was the time of outdoor walks around the hospital grounds of Kernan with Mike.

Strongly support the need for thinking skills therapy, and compensatory strategies for memory. Your loved one may claim to be completely normal and may want to go home. However, they still have remaining problems.

Your loved one's own assessment of their abilities is probably not accurate. Make sure that you check with the attending physician and treatment team concerning any restrictions (driving, drinking, etc…) *This may have been when I refused to take my meals in the dining hall with the rest of the patients. I remember that I felt like I had nothing in common with them, and they irritated me for some reason.*

3. Frequently discuss daily activities with your loved one to expand their memory.

Encouraging them to remember detail is excellent, so is journalizing. *My family always wanted to hear me tell about my daily activities, including what I had been served at meal time.*

4. Help them fill in gaps for the very common memory loss (amnesia) around the accident. *They kept telling me about the accident, but it didn't mean anything to me.*

5. Talk in a normal fashion. Simplifying your language is no longer necessary. However, your loved one is apt to be literal minded. They will not "get" subtleties or innuendo. Misunderstandings are very common. *I am still very much like this, and it can hamper normal adult conversation.*

Level VIII:

It was probably at this stage that I was released from Kernan to Mike's care.

1. Participate with the person in familiar activities in order to help them become aware of some of their limitations. Point out alternative ways to accomplish goals. Always be non-critical and non-competitive.

2. Help your loved one develop the very useful and important habit of note taking. This is to compensate for memory difficulties, which are apt to be permanent.

3. Anger and frustration are common with brain injury. Help your loved one cope by talking it over. Discussing what frustrates them and makes them angry will provide opportunities to develop new behaviors.

4. Encourage your loved one to talk to you about how they feel about going home. It is normal to be depressed or nervous. Do not tell them that they have no reason to feel this way. Also, freely talk about community reactions, especially if disabilities are evident.

5. Maintain a hopeful, yet realistic attitude. Understand that learning to cope with permanent cognitive limitations takes months or years.

Levels IX and X:

Levels IX and X describe the current me.

I picked up the pretty, green pendant that matched my earrings and draped it around my neck. As I strode across my room attempting to fasten it at the back of my neck, I could feel my clumsy fingers fail to do it. Instead of asking for assistance from my husband, I stubbornly turned and strode back across the room, still struggling. My continued failure to clasp the pendant became unbearable to me. I stamped my feet, uttered an expletive, and burst into tears when my husband chided me for misbehaving and scaring the dog. I threw the necklace onto my dresser and continued to prepare to go to the office seething with anger and resentment.

Family members need to anticipate problems and take steps to prevent them from escalating. It is important to allow your loved one independence, but not at the cost of their self-esteem. The person with brain injury may be a challenge to your reserves of patience. Try hard to be very gentle but firm when you must correct their behavior. The best tool available to teach your loved one proper behavior is your example. Be a role model for the one with brain injury. Do not exhibit shock or dismay when your family member is depressed or irritable. Instead, invite your loved one to use you as a sounding board. The one with brain injury is not always looking for solutions, but is invariably comforted by an interested, non-critical listener.

I was at the gym. The shower portion of the women's locker room was closed for construction. After my workout, I entered one of the two "family" locker/shower/changing rooms and locked the door. In the midst of my shower, there was a pounding on the door, shouting, and the door handle was rattled. I yelled out that the room was occupied, to no avail. The loud, rude male continued jiggling the handle and pounding on the door. I quickly rinsed off, barely dried myself, threw some clothing on, and gingerly opened the door. I was greeted by the angry male, his wheel chaired wife, and a staff member. The staff member was unable to calm the situation, so I was treated to more verbal abuse by the man and also by his disabled wife. I was horribly shaken, but managed to make my way upstairs to the reception desk. At this point, I could not contain my emotions any longer. Staff gathered behind the counter, and curious members stopped to stare as I allowed the full extent of my wrath out (I threw a tantrum.) This incident describes one of my worst experiences when trying to achieve independence. If my caregiver had been present, he could have helped me to make a more appropriate choice to avoid the ugly scene (shower at home.)

Sources: <u>Living with Brain Injury - A Guide for Families</u>, Richard C. Senelick, MD and Cathy E. Ryan, MA, CCC-SLP. Websites: <u>www.waiting.com</u>, <u>www.caregiver-information.com</u>, <u>www.learningservices.com</u>, <u>www.traumaticbraininjury.com</u>.

What Does It All Mean...

"If I had a day that I could give you, I'd give to you a day just like today."
-John Denver

When I started writing this book in the spring of 2005, it was a result of contact with the Helen Keller Foundation. A colleague at BIAM gave me a flier announcing a writing contest for possible inclusion in an anthology. The foundation was asking for 3000-word memoirs about overcoming disability. I wrote an essay called, "To the Summit or Bust," and submitted the manuscript. A few months later I was excited to learn that my essay had been selected for inclusion in the anthology. The resulting book was published and released on August 1, 2008, and is entitled, <u>Reading Lips and Other Ways to Overcome a Disability</u>, edited by Diane Scharper and Philip Scharper, Jr., M.D. I am honored to be among the twenty-nine different authors presented in the pages of the book.

Helen Keller's riveting story is about a woman's triumph over massive obstacles, owing to her high intelligence, her unquenchable determination, her incredible valor, and with tremendous support from family and friends. The book contains twenty-nine Helen Keller-like stories that will inspire anyone to keep trying, in the midst of great difficulties. The acceptance of my manuscript inspired me to write an autobiographical account of my recovery from brain injury, of which the 3000-word memoir is an excerpt. "To the Summit or Bust" became a memoir within a memoir. Thanks to God, I had not lost all of me and the letter of acceptance from the foundation was tangible proof. My hope is that you will notice the maturation process that I have been going through since my accident. It is the reason why A) I have arranged the book chronologically, according to what I wrote first to what I wrote last, B) I have not rewritten anything from four years ago, even though my skills have improved, and C) I let my words bear witness to the real possibility of human growth (without hormones.) In addition, I want you to note some of the requirements for a good recovery from brain injury, and lastly, I would like you to understand that recovery is a continuous process.

My story commences with a haunting visit from my deceased mother because she is the one who told me to return to life. The vision is still very real to me and it marks the beginning of my increased spirituality. What happens to us after we die? It is no longer a mystery to me. The woman in the garden was young, healthy, and pretty – a very different vision from the one I have from her last day of life. My mother, with whom I had an estranged relationship for years, was the one who gave me life in the beginning and then gave it back to me when it was almost lost. When I think about her now, it is with clemency. The clarifying revelation I experienced was both comforting and illuminating.

During my time of darkness, I was also consoled by a soothing male voice. On more than one occasion, he whispered in my ear, "Your pain won't last forever. You'll be okay. Don't give up." Upon waking, I not only asked my husband about my mother, but I also told him that I was with Jesus. The feelings of joy and wonder with which I emerged from coma are still with me and are responsible for enabling me to successfully crawl out of the darkness of depression occasionally. Now you know the source of my inner voice. It is important for you to believe that the inner voice is in you, too, no matter what the name of your source.

While reading my book, you may have noticed a child's voice – simple, straightforward expressions, single-mindedness, literal mindedness, immaturity, self-involved thought processes, petulance, and hero worship. You are not wrong to conclude that the author needs to grow up. My husband tells me and everyone else that one of the most startling aspects of my emergence from coma was my "little girl" voice. To hear him describe it is both heart-breaking and fascinating. Emergence from coma is a long process that can last days, weeks, months, or years, depending upon the unique aspects of the individual. In other words, it is not an on/off switch. Furthermore, if the brain injury is severe enough, the patient starts from the very beginning of their existence. They mature through infancy, through childhood, through adolescence, and into adulthood. For these reasons, it is not surprising that I can sometimes sound like an adolescent. My husband tells me that I remind him of a young adult, now, and we laugh about it. To be a caregiver is the hardest job of all. All of you, who are parents, think about it. Is it not true? Can you imagine what it is like to "bring up" your spouse? Mike wrote me this short story that illustrates my point beautifully; I treasure it.

The Ant and the Twig

A very long time ago there was an ant. The young ant was born, as most ants are, very high up on an old

*and worn mountain. As the ant grew, he had heard
of a wonderful valley down below. Up on the old
mountain it was chilly all the time. There was little
to eat and life, as it was, was dismal. He had heard
that the valley was paradise. Ants were fat and happy
down there. It was always warm in the valley. There
was plenty to eat in the valley. It was heaven.*

*The problem was that the valley was over 50 miles
away. Many who tried to make it to the valley had
a tragic end. Those who walked down were either
crushed under foot or somehow just lost their way.
Some tried to go down the very tiny little stream that
was up on the old mountain. The wise ants told them
that the stream was the only way. The problem was,
many who believed in using the stream perished on
the journey and never made it to the valley. Some just
jumped in the stream, floated, got water logged, or got
lost on a tributary and ended up on land no closer to
the valley than they started. Some jumped in groups
onto big safe logs and tried to make it to the valley.
Their trip was often bumpy and they would fall off.
Other times the log was too big and got stuck in the
stream and the ants would either spend their entire
lives on the log or they would get off the log and be lost.*

*The young ant decided he would look around, and
found a little twig that had fallen off an old maple tree.
He carried the little twig on his back, gently set it on*

the stream, and held on to it, and off they went down the stream. The little twig floated swiftly down the stream and ant quickly learned how to guide it down the stream safely. What a great idea. They were on their way to the valley and to his surprise, it was fun.

Now, 50 miles is a long way. Imagine how long it is to a little twig and an ant. The stream grew wider as time went on. There were rapid, fast days and there were calm, lazy days. It was less and less chilly as they went on. Time went by quickly and they knew they were going in the right direction towards the valley, but it was hard to tell how much longer it would be before they got to the valley. The young ant remembered the wise ants telling him the trip is long for some and short for others. You will know the valley when you get there.

Sometimes the ant would guide the twig to the shore. He would carry the twig to the shore so it could dry off. He would walk around on land again to get his legs back in shape. One day, after walking around he couldn't find the twig where he had left it. He was about as upset as an ant can get. After desperately searching, he found the little twig. It had been rammed by one of those giant logs full of ants. It was bent and damaged. He knew it wasn't completely broken after sitting next to it and watching it for a while. He remembered the wise ants telling him that *twigs need moisture to survive. So he slipped into the stream to carry back moisture for the twig. It was then he realized that he couldn't swim. He couldn't even float. He almost drowned. Oh, how he needed that twig. Well, he taught himself to float, a little. Every day he would get a little moisture and carry it to the twig and the twig got stronger and stronger.*

Finally, they both decided that the twig was strong enough to continue the journey, the journey to the valley, the journey to paradise, the journey to heaven. So the ant gently lifted the twig into the stream, grabbed on and off they went. Early on, the ant did the guiding down the stream. As time went on, the twig started getting even stronger than before and they took turns guiding.

Now, word got out, as it often does with ants, about the little ant and how he patiently brought moisture to the twig, and how the twig grew stronger and stronger. But the ant would just shake his head and say, "I will never make it to the valley without that twig."

They were last seen on their journey floating down the stream on their way, for sure, to the valley...together.

To Eileen from Mike with love. October 3, 2007.

What does it take to make as good a recovery from brain injury as possible? I have tried to make it clear throughout this book.

- **Support** – Someone to watch over you; someone to nurture you; someone to guide you; someone to protect you; someone to love you just as you are; someone who needs you, too. A group or an organization who understands, who can provide encouragement, who has helpful ideas and resources, and who can be your advocate.

Vulnerability is the hallmark of brain injury. A survivor can be rendered almost helpless, even though he or she may have been wise, strong, and independent pre-injury.

Suddenly, their defenses are down, their judgment is impaired, they may have post-traumatic stress, their employability is negligible, and they may have mobility challenges. It is difficult to accept, but an adult brain injury survivor may be temporarily childlike. In a worst-case scenario, the state may persist for a lifetime. Imagine what catastrophes can happen to vulnerable individuals without support. The best resources are: family, friends, spiritual communities, professional counselors, support groups, and organizations dedicated to brain injury and its effects.

- **Determination** – Enough inner strength to keep you going when obstacles appear; a strong desire to be better than you are today; the fortitude to accept challenges; the character to finish the job.

Never underestimate the value of determination. The road to recovery is long, uphill, and un-paved; you will encounter obstacles – that's a given. It is so easy to become discouraged. Just remember, that you are worth whatever is required to overcome your disability in order to keep moving forward. Listen to your inner voice; it will never mislead you, because it has **only your** best interests at heart. If the rewards are desirable, do not shy away from the challenges to obtain them. You may be pleasantly surprised by your forgotten abilities. Every task that you complete becomes part of a growing collection of your successes. Pat yourself on the back once in a while.

- **Faith** – In God, the one who you acknowledge knows better than you; in yourself, because you believe in your value as a human being; in others, because you like being in their company, and they can aid in your recovery.

To believe in something is like being the kitten after a toy on a string. There is an irresistible desire to leap forward. Neither circumstances nor depression can keep you down very long if you believe in yourself, a divine presence, and other people. Keep in mind that you represent the best of God's creation, and that He is extremely proud of you, just like any loving parent would be. He will not let you down, so keep in touch with Him through your inner voice.

- **Opportunity** – For rehabilitation, both formal and informal; for employment, for both income and self-esteem; for loving relationships, both romantic and familial; for counseling, both spiritual and secular, to help you discover your own inner strength.

Given enough time and patience, even a tortoise will reach the finish line. Brain injury survivors are a team of tortoises but we are still viable participants in life. Don't bet against us. Remember how disengaged from her environment Helen Keller was? Communication was the key that unlocked the world to her. Once that happened, she eventually graduated from college *Cum Laude* and learned to speak seven languages! The biggest losers were the ones who bet against her.

Rehabilitation is one of the keys that will open up the world to survivors. It exists in our society in many different forms, including the one I am currently engaged in – college. However, opportunity is not always present. Medical insurance will pay for a survivor's "traditional" rehabilitation for a time, but it is generally terminated not at the will of a survivor or their family. Insurance companies will pay for a limited number of rehab sessions according to a preset "standard." This ludicrous habit assumes that all brain injuries are alike when they are actually as individual as fingerprints. Contrary to expectation, the insurance companies are not always to blame, though. Sometimes the blame lies with the survivor, the family, or with society. If any of the following factors is missing, the road to rehab can be barricaded: motivation, guidance, transportation, insurance, and money. What is society's role? How about showing more patience, tolerance, and understanding when encountering one of us on the public transportation system? How about donating some of your time as a volunteer to our cause with an organization like the Brain Injury Association of Maryland? How about not objecting when the state or federal government wants to spend a little money on us? It is our government, too. How about offering us reasonable employment even though we are different?

The toughest issue, by far, that we deal with is relationships – maintaining them post-injury or starting them post-injury. It is the most popular topic of conversation at our support group meetings. Too many marriages end in divorce when one spouse acquires a brain injury. Finding a mate or a date is a huge challenge for us and fulfilling our duties as parents, as grandparents, or as siblings presents unexpected difficulties. We are changed permanently upon acquisition of a brain injury and sometimes those changes wreak havoc in our relationships. Our spouses chose to dedicate themselves to someone who no longer exists. Therefore, unless the new person possesses qualities that are equally as attractive as the originals, the love relationship can expire. Our children attached themselves to someone who no longer exists. How can they be expected to feel obliged to take advice from a stranger? Furthermore, if their beloved mother or father is changed, will that not result in insecurity for the youngsters? Our siblings grew up with someone who no longer exists. A lifetime of bonding can be broken by brain injury.

- **Forgiveness** – Anyone you blame for your brain injury -- God, yourself, and others. You will rid yourself of one more impediment to getting on with your life.

I wrote the following essay for my first college class. My professor liked it; I hope you do, too.

Forgiveness

Forgiveness is empathy. Try to identify with the other person or situation. It is very hard to do and requires an open mind. Someone you know and care about may be cross with you, and speaks to you impatiently. Can you find it in your heart to ignore the anger

inside you, and instead, gently ask if the other person is okay? Perhaps you can ask a question or two about their situation instead of focusing on your own feelings.

Forgiveness is courage. Someone is screaming at you. Their face is full of hatred, and their words feel like needles. Are you brave enough to not run away? Can you withstand the pain of listening to them? If so, self esteem is your reward.

Forgiveness is genuineness. Imagining it, theorizing about it, or wishing for it is not enough. Genuineness is to forgiveness what baking is to bread. Forgiveness is incomplete unless you actually do it.

Forgiveness is satisfying. I was badly injured because someone hit my vehicle head-on with their truck when they were distracted. For many stress-filled months I thought of nothing else but the unfairness of it all. One day I decided to forgive him. From that day on, I was free of stress, agitation, and sleeplessness. I was finally able to sit back and relax.

Forgiveness is entirely subjective. It is something that we do for ourselves. The act of sincere forgiveness enables us to go on with the rest of our lives.

Forgiveness does not require the other person to know about it or to be grateful. It can be one's own secret pleasure.

Forgiveness is lavender for the soul.

I have learned so much about me and about other BI survivors during the past nine years. Co-facilitating a brain injury support group has been both gratifying and highly educational. I will share with you an interesting observation of us that I have made. We can be categorized in basically two groups, no matter what our level of recovery. In addition, we can start in one group and move into another, or we can shift back and forth between groups more than once. It is also interesting to answer the following questions.

Who am I? Who are you?

	Total Independence Now (TIN	Boss of Leisure (BOL)
Attributes	•Decision Maker •Desiring pace/tranquility •Avoiding stress through organization	•Decision maker •Desiring peace/tranquility •Avoiding stress through inactivity
Benefits	•Doing it yourself •Self-Knowledge •Control of one's own life/independence	•Having someone do it for you •More leisure time •Less stress and fatigue •More peace and tranquility
Hazards	•Stress •Fatigue •Aggressiveness •Vulnerability	•Loss of control of one's •own life/dependence •Procrastination •Deferred maturation •Vulnerability

What about tomorrow?

It is difficult for me to answer such a question because I tend to live for today, post-injury. However, I will take a moment to talk about the challenges that I may still have to face in the future. The symptoms that still trouble me primarily are:

- A slower processing speed

- Reduced capacity

- Loss of self

- Uneven emotions

Slower Processing Speed

This one is the culprit for much of my misunderstandings. It is not possible for others to slow down to my speed and I cannot speed up to theirs. Consequently, I will continue to ask for the indulgence of others to repeat essential details and I must disregard what is not important. I also need to find a way to avoid being hurt when chastised by loved ones due to misunderstandings. I will continue to read directions more than once and to not rush through any unfamiliar activity. At school, I will continue to use the syllabus to work ahead of the lecture and to take extra time for tests. Psychologically, I need to protect my self-esteem by not feeling ashamed of my slowness. Instead, I will continue to celebrate my successes so that I can feel proud of my ability to complete projects.

Reduced Capacity

The meaning of this symptom is that I can complete a smaller list of tasks than I could pre-injury, and it is a direct result of having a slower processing speed. The potential for sudden, overwhelming fatigue is also a factor. The strategy that I have worked out for this challenge is to simply take on only what I can accomplish in a reasonable amount of time. The hardest part is to be disciplined and to resist saying "yes" to everything that is asked of me. If I become employed again, the job must entail a work load that I am certain to be able to accomplish. I must remember to avoid taking on too big a challenge.

Loss of Self

This one scares me the most because it can lead to loneliness and depression. I have to find a way to let go of my old identity and embrace my new one. I am hopeful that if I continue to look for and to find new strengths and abilities in the new Eileen, I will stop looking for the old Eileen. Over time, I expect to become comfortable with the new me. Loss of self is the one aspect of brain injury that I suspect will not last forever.

Uneven Emotions

This symptom is the one that frustrates my loved ones and embarrasses me. It is also the one for which I still need professional counseling the most. When I tell Dr. Hopkins that he is my *Prozac*, it is a statement of fact. Regular counseling does help to keep me stable. On my own, I need to call on my inner voice to guide me.

You may call it prayer or meditation, but it is still a coping skill that works. When I perceive that others are being unkind, I must not add to my suffering by dwelling on it. Learning to let go is a skill that I am certain will require a lifetime of practice.

What I will mention last is the most important part of being human, with, or without a brain injury – personal relationships. I need to remember to not throw away the relationship when I am ignoring a loved one's bad behavior. When the bad behavior is over, I have to remember to show my enjoyment of good behavior. In other words, don't let resentment grow so large, that it blocks the sun. I can't thrive without love.

Recovery has only a beginning but no end. While it may be true to say that two years post-injury you will feel more like yourself (I know this from personal experience), it is *not* true to say that you are as good as you are going to get. When I consider how I was at the two year anniversary of my accident, and compare it to how I am now, I am gratified and grateful for my progress. Developmentally, I am much less childlike. Even my counselor lets me know that I have matured cognitively and socially since we have known each other.

On a sparkling day in early autumn, it happened. I was working through my list of chores, feeling thankful for the enhancement of the color green in the sun and for the fresh scent delivered by the brisk breeze. The date on the calendar caught my attention; it was October 3rd, and my ninth birthday. I marveled at my lack of apprehension. For close to a decade, this date had always been a day full of anxiety. Indeed, the approach of Fall-like days had been times of foreboding for me. But on this day, nine years post-trauma, the sense of dread was absent. I still felt disturbed by the knowledge of the seriousness of the event and the days that followed, but the usual tears did not come. Instead, I felt energized and excited by the revelation that God had given me a second life and that He must believe in me. It was then I realized the true meaning of the motor vehicle collision. It was the day that negativity died.

On April 9, 2010, I stood before an audience of 200 to 300 people giving an opening keynote address. The occasion was the annual two-day educational conference presented by the Brain Injury Association of Maryland. The conference is a comprehensive collection of speakers and presenters who offer information, support, and inspiration to survivors, caregivers, and professionals.

When Diane Triplett asked me to be a keynote speaker in June 2009, I was honored. I was also scared that I would not be able to deliver an address worthy to be among the ones I had heard over the years. I started writing my speech in January, and over the next three months, it went through many revisions. It was the subject of several of my meetings with Bill Hopkins during that time, and his advice was invaluable.

The name of my speech was "Legacies and Possibilities." It was a one hour and fifteen minute address that included time for questions and answers. I was gratified when my listeners occasionally interrupted me to ask a question even before I finished speaking. They showed genuine interest, and their questions were thoughtful and intelligent.

My PowerPoint presentation started with a picture of Helen Keller. She was a real American hero, and her story illustrates that her disability was what she made of it and society's evaluation was not a factor. This is a powerful message for persons with any disability, not just brain injury, and I wanted my people to hear it. My speech continued on a positive note but did not ignore the challenges of living with brain injury. I discussed my experiences with post secondary education and then went on to the Kubler-Ross five stages of grief. The audience reacted with murmurs and comments indicating that this was part of their world, too. I informed the group that I believe that I reached stage 5, acceptance, in October 2009, upon the ninth anniversary of the motor vehicle accident.

The most important part of my speech came near the end, when I listed for my audience all the gifts with injury that I have received. That was how I illustrated that I am better with a brain injury than without and that I would not trade my disability for anything. There was a slight gasp and then silence when I announced that the brain injury is probably the best thing that could have happened to me.

I ended my speech with a question for the audience, "What do you want your legacy to be?" I want mine to be, *I never lost what I love the most; I just gained the most of what I love.*

If success is measured in self-confidence, happiness, and satisfaction, then I have achieved it. I began my journey to healing over nine years ago, full of anger, resentment, and grief. Today, the many blessings that are mine because of the brain injury bring me incredible joy. I hope that my experience displays the elasticity of the human brain and the unquenchable human spirit. I believe in God; I believe in me; I believe in you. Together, we are the can-do crew.

Resources...

Brain Injury Association of Maryland, Inc.
2200 Kernan Drive
Baltimore, MD 21207
(410) 448-2924
(800) 221-6443
www.biamd.org

William Hopkins, Ph.D.
Licensed Psychologist
Carroll Counseling Center
1380 Progress Way, Suite 101
Eldersburg, MD 21784
www.carrollcounseling.com

Joyce Sebian
Specialist for Students with Disability
Carroll Community College
1601 Washington Road
Westminster, MD 21157
www.carrollcc.edu

Carnell Cooper, M.D.
Associate Professor of Surgery
University of Maryland Medical Center
22 S. Greene Street
Baltimore, MD 21201
www.umm.edu/shocktrauma

Michael Makley, M.D.
Director, TBI Unit
Kernan Orthopaedics and Rehabilitation
2200 Kernan Drive
Baltimore, MD 21207
www.kernan.org

Navin Singh, M.D.
Ivy Plastic Surgery Associates
5454 Wisconsin Ave., Suite 1710
Chevy Chase, MD 20815
www.ivyplasticsurgery.com

Remy H. Blanchaert Jr., DDS, M.D.
Oral and Maxillofacial Surgery Associates
1919 N. Webb Road
Wichita, KS 67206-3405
www.wichitaoms.com

Andrew W. Eglseder, M.D.
Associate Professor Orthopaedic Surgery
University of Maryland Medical Center
22 S. Greene Street
Baltimore, MD 21201
www.umm.edu/shocktrauma

Michael A. Freedman, P.A.
10019 Reisterstown Road
Suite 204
Owings Mills, MD 21117
www.maflaw.com

Reese Volunteer Fire Company
Station 9
1745 Baltimore Blvd.
Westminster, MD 21157
www.reesevfc.org

About the Author...

Eileen Rudnick was born in Montreal, Canada and emigrated to the U.S. in 1965. She is married to Michael Rudnick LPN, her spouse of 39 years. They have two grown children and two grandchildren and currently live in Carroll County, Maryland.

Eileen was an accountant for many years before the traffic accident that changed her life in 2000. She is currently a student at Carroll Community College with a 4.0 GPA and a member of two different honor societies - Phi Theta Kappa and Delta Alpha Pi. Eileen also spends some of her time tutoring her classmates in math and writing. She has been writing since she was eight years old and is seeking a degree in English.

After her rehabilitation at Kernan Hospital in Woodlawn, Eileen returned to volunteer in the office of the Brain Injury Association of Maryland (www.biamd.org) She is also the co-facilitator of a brain injury support group in Eldersburg with her husband.

The anthology <u>Reading Lips and Other Ways to Overcome a Disability</u>, published by Apprentice House, contains a memoir by Eileen called, "To the Summit or Bust." She was also the subject of the article, "Sustaining Spirit," in the June 2009 issue of Baltimore Magazine (www.baltimormagazine.net). Eileen was interviewed on WCBM talk radio on Sept. 5th, 2009 (www.womantalklive.com)

Today, Eileen is a brain injury survivor advocate and a motivational speaker on their behalf. Contact Eileen via eileen.rudnick@gmail.com.

The future of publishing...today!

Apprentice House is the country's only campus-based, student-staffed book publishing company. Directed by professors and industry professionals, it is a nonprofit activity of the Communication Department at Loyola University Maryland.

Using state-of-the-art technology and an experiential learning model of education, Apprentice House publishes books in untraditional ways. This dual responsibility as publishers and educators creates an unprecedented collaborative environment among faculty and students, while teaching tomorrow's editors, designers, and marketers.

Outside of class, progress on book projects is carried forth by the AH Book Publishing Club, a co-curricular campus organization supported by Loyola University Maryland's Office of Student Activities.

Student Project Team for *The Glass Between Us:*
    Storm Sebastian, '11

Eclectic and provocative, Apprentice House titles intend to entertain as well as spark dialogue on a variety of topics. Financial contributions to sustain the press's work are welcomed. Contributions are tax deductible to the fullest extent allowed by the IRS.

To learn more about Apprentice House books or to obtain submission guidelines, please visit www.ApprenticeHouse.com.

Apprentice House
Communication Department
Loyola University Maryland
4501 N. Charles Street
Baltimore, MD 21210
Ph: 410-617-5265 • Fax: 410-617-2198
info@apprenticehouse.com